BRADY

Trauma Update for the Emergency Medical Technician

Continuing Education Series

Richard L. Judd, Ph.D., Series Editor

Hazardous Material Exposure:
Emergency Response and Patient Care

Jonathan Borak, M.D.
Michael Callan
William Abbott

Emergency Services Stress

Jeff Mitchell, Ph.D.

Trauma Update for the Emergency Medical Technician

Kimball Maull, M.D.
Jackie Kirby, R.N., M.S.N., C.C.R.N.
Dennis Rowe, EMT-P

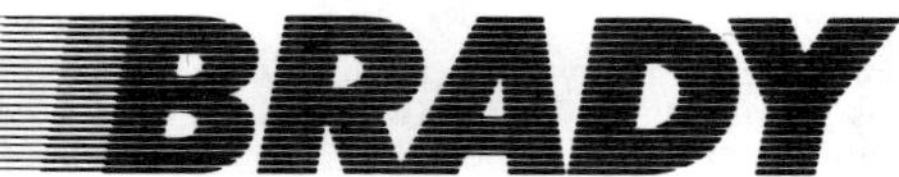

TRAUMA UPDATE FOR THE EMERGENCY MEDICAL TECHNICIAN

Kimball I. Maull, M.D.
Professor and Chairman
Department of Surgery
University of Tennessee Medical Center at Knoxville

Jackie Kirby, R.N., M.S.N. C.C.R.N.
Trauma Nurse Coordinator
Department of Surgery
University of Tennessee Medical Center at Knoxville

Dennis Rowe, EMT–P
Flight Paramedic and Educational Coordinator
Lifestar Aeromedical Service
University of Tennessee Medical Center at Knoxville

Editors

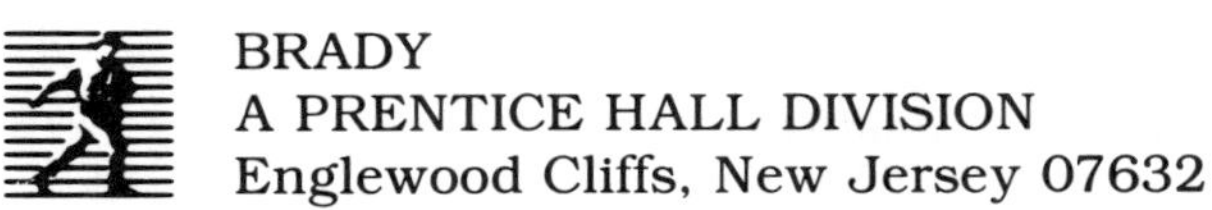
BRADY
A PRENTICE HALL DIVISION
Englewood Cliffs, New Jersey 07632

Maull, Kimball I. (Kimball Ivan), 1942–
Trauma update for the emergency medical technician / Kimball Maull, editor, Dennis Rowe, editor, Jackie Kirby, editor.
p. cm. — (Continuing education series)
Includes index.
ISBN 0-89303-889-X
1. Emergency medicine. 2. Medical emergencies. 3. Emergency medical technicians. I. Rowe, Dennis. II. Kirby, Jackie M. III. Title. IV. Series: Continuing education series (Englewood Cliffs, N.J.)
[DNLM: 1. Emergencies. 2. Emergency Medical Services. 3. Emergency Mecical Technicians. 4. Wounds and Injuries—therapy. WO 700 M449t]
RC86.7.M385 1992
616.02'5—dc20
DNLM/DLC
for Library of Congress 91–40778
CIP

Editorial/production supervision: **Marcia Krefetz**
Acquisitions Editor: **Natalie Anderson**
Interior design: **Ed Jones**
Cover design: **Joe Di Domenico**
Manufacturing Buyer: **Ed O'Dougherty**
Prepress Buyer: **Ilene Levy**
Editorial Assistant: **Louise Fullam**
Production Assistant: **Bunnie Neuman**

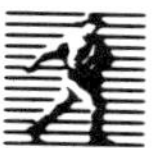

A Division of Simon & Schuster
Englewood Cliffs, New Jersey 07632

Notice: The author and the publisher of this book have taken care to make certain that the equipment, doses of drugs and schedules of treatment are correct and compatible with the standards generally accepted at the time of publication. Nevertheless, as new information becomes available, changes in treatment and in the use of equipment and drugs become necessary. The reader is advised to carefully consult the instruction and information material included in the package insert of each drug or therapeutic agent, piece of equipment or device before administration. This advice is especially important when using new or infrequently used drugs. No endorsement by the American Heart Association or any of its committees is stated or implied, nor is there any suggested warranty of performance during the American Heart Association Advanced Cardiac Life Support Course. Prehospital Care Providers are warned that use of any drugs or techniques must be authorized by their medical advisor, in accord with local laws and regulations. The publisher disclaims any liability, loss, injury, or damage incurred as a consequence, directly or indirectly, of the use and applicationn of any of the contents of this book.

Printed in the United States of America
10 9 8 7 6 5 4 3 2 1

ISBN 0-89303-889-X

Prentice-Hall International (UK) Limited, *London*
Prentice-Hall of Australia Pty. Limited, *Sydney*
Prentice-Hall Canada Inc., *Toronto*
Prentice-Hall Hispanoamericana, S.A., *Mexico*
Prentice-Hall of Indian Private Limited, *New Delhi*
Prentice-Hall of Japan, Inc., *Tokyo*
Simon & Schuster Asia Pte. Ltd., *Singapore*
Editora Prentice-Hall do Brasil, Ltda., *Rio de Janeiro*

Contributing Authors

University of Tennessee Medical Center at Knoxville

Hobart E. Akin, MD
Assistant Professor of Surgery
Abdominal Injuries

Darrell Brackett, EMT–P
Flight Paramedic, Lifestar
Spine and Spinal Cord Trauma

R. Christopher Brooks, MD
Emergency Physician
Environmental Hazards

Larry Hardison, RN, EMT–P
Staff Nurse, Trauma Intensive Care Unit
Head Trauma

Rick Harrington, EMT–P
Flight Paramedic, Lifestar
Upper Airway Management and Ventilation
Mass Casualties
Aircraft Crashes

Rhea Waring Hart, FN, EMT-A, CEN
Abdominal Injuries

Walter Idol, EMT–P
Flight Paramedic, Lifestar
Extrication, Packaging, and Transport

Glenn E. Jeffries, MD
Chief, Division of Orthopedic Surgery
Extremity Trauma

Jackie Kirby, RN, MSN, CCRN
Trauma Nurse Coordinator
Department of Surgery
Kinematics

Les Lougheed, EMT–P
Flight Paramedic, Lifestar
Basic Water Rescue
Cave and Mine Rescue

Kimball I. Maull, MD
Professor and Chairman, Department of Surgery
Trauma in Pregnancy

J. Tucker Montgomery, MD, JD
Emergency Physician
Medicolegal Aspects of Prehospital Care

Henry S. Nelson, Jr., MD
Assistant Professor of Surgery
Shock

Dan E. Norman
Chief Pilot and Director of Operations, Lifestar
Aircraft Crashes

Randall E. Pedigo, MD
Assistant Professor of Surgery
Thoracic Injuries

Dennis Rowe, EMT–P
Flight Paramedic, Lifestar
Initial Evaluation
Extremity Trauma
Pediatric Trauma

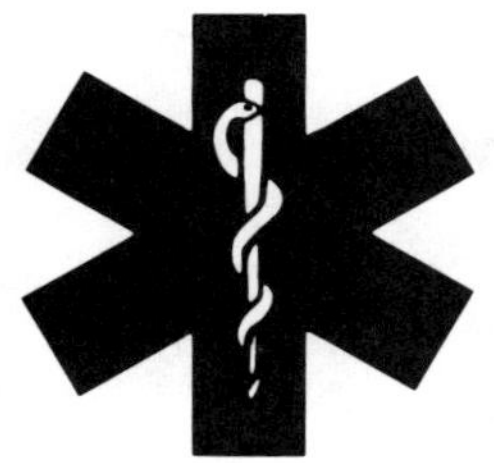

Contents

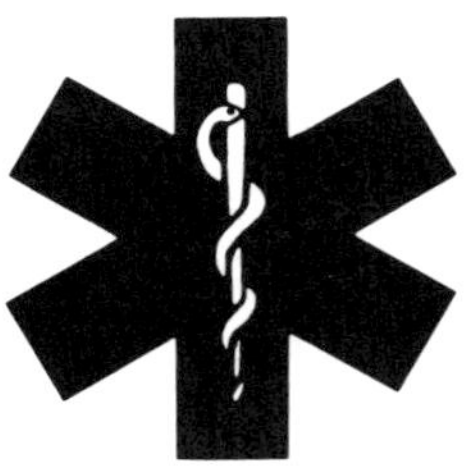

Foreword

There have been great strides in the delivery of emergency medical service since President Nixon signed the law creating emergency medical systems nationwide in 1973. The backbone of these systems is the emergency medical technicians who provide service to ill or injured patients on a daily basis. The altruism of those men and women who venture out day or night to the scene of an incident, ready to tend to an unknown patient, is the essence of emergency medical technology.

The desire to help others in an emergency is clearly recorded in the earliest writings in history. However, systems for delivering trauma care were not well organized until the time of Baron Dominique-Jean Larrey, Napoleon's surgeon. Larrey recognized that time was most important in the survival of soldiers injured in battle. He developed a system of small, horse-drawn carriages with emergency medical corpsmen that would dart into the field of battle, collect a wounded soldier, and take him to an aid station where care was delivered by surgeons.

These principles have withstood the test of time and have been applied over and over again in our own century—in the two world wars, the Korean conflict, Vietnam, and the Faulklands. The only changes have been in the technology and the type of transportation used. Horse-drawn ambulances were replaced by motor ambulances, and ultimately by helicopters.

The fundamental component of this system has always been the corpsmen or emergency medical technicians who brave the adversity of the battlefield to deliver care to an injured patient.

Emergency trauma care in the civilian arena is very similar. Training and education are essential if the emergency medical technician is to achieve a favorable outcome for the patient. Initially, the excitement of being dispatched to an emergency scene may repress any feelings of inadequacy or fear. At the scene, however, it is the depth and intensity of the technician's training, along with confidence in his or her skills, that will determine the effectiveness of resuscitative efforts.

This book will be of great use to those ememgency medical technicians who wish to be fully prepared for all emergencies they may encounter in the field. It provides not only the basic skills of resuscitation, but also an understanding of the principles underlying these techniques. Both are essential if the technician is to become a sound practitioner. Each chapter in this text has a set of objectives to guide the reader. Throughout the text are figures that illustrate key principles. The text is augmented by an Instructor's Manual, which includes questions directly derived from the material covered in the chapter. The answer list and accompanying discussion will help the instructor evaluate what the reader has learned.

The authors have incorporated practical information in a well-organized text. The result is a comprehensive, up-to-date review of field trauma care that also addresses the unique problems that emergency technicians often encounter. Finally, the text includes a chapter on medical-legal issues that should be required reading for every emergency medical technician.

This text should become a friend and companion for those dedicated people who venture forth in adverse circumstances to render aid and assistance to the unfortunate patient who has been injured.

Lenworth M. Jacobs, M.D. M.P.H., F.A.C.S.

Director, Trauma Program/Emergency Medicine,
Hartford Hospital
Professor of Surgery,
University of Connecticut School of Medicine

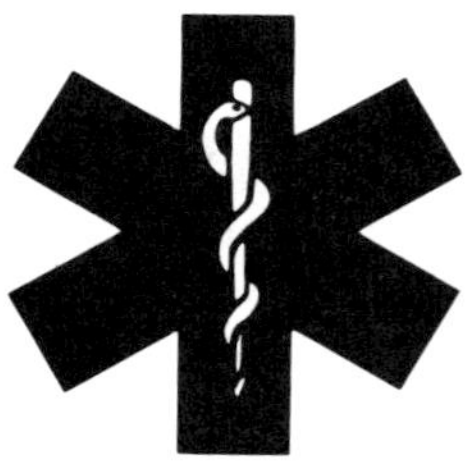

Preface

Trauma is a disease—a disease of injuries that may be incurred accidentally, inflicted intentionally by others, or self-inflicted. Trauma is the most important, most expensive, and most tragic health problem in the United States, costing more years of life than cancer and heart disease combined. The cost of trauma is now estimated to exceed 180 billion dollars annually, and it increases each year. Trauma is the leading cause of death in people between the ages of 1 and 40. Each year 60 to 70 million people are injured. Thus, trauma affects approximately one-fourth of the population every year, killing 150,000, temporarily disabling 11 million, and permanently disabling approximately 470,000. Although trauma can strike at any age, it is primarily a disease of the young, and the cost to society is great for the non–wage earner who becomes dependent on society for his or her maintenance.

The outcome of an injury depends on a finite number of factors. These trauma outcome determinants are of two general types: those over which health care providers have no control, and those over which they do have control. In the latter case, attention to optimal care principles can make a difference between life and death, or between full recovery and lasting disability.

The principle outcome determinant is *severity of injury*. Approximately 50 percent of trauma victims die within minutes. Since injury severity cannot be lessened after the fact, trauma prevention is the only means of dealing with this large number of deaths. Trauma prevention has even broader implications for major disabling injuries.

Age of the patient is the second determinant over which the health care provider has no control. It is widely known that given injuries of equal severity, the elderly patient will more likely have an adverse outcome than the young adult. Age is indirectly related to the third trauma-outcome determinant, *preexisting medical condition of the patient.* If two 40-year-olds sustained injuries of equal severity, and one was in good health and the other had juvenile-onset diabetes mellitus, hypertension, and a smoking habit, the latter individual would more likely have an adverse outcome. None of these three trauma-outcome determinants are directly amenable to modification by an optimal emergency medical service (EMS) system.

The fourth trauma-outcome determinant—and the first over which health care providers have control—is *time.* As Dr. R Adams Cowley noted in the early 1960s, reducing the time between trauma and definitive care improves the chances for survival. He identified the first 60 minutes after trauma as the ''golden hour'' and cautioned EMS providers that for every additional 60 minutes that transpires beyond the Golden Hour, mortality rises threefold. For example, if a person with a ruptured spleen who is treated within 60 minutes of the injury has a 1-in-10 chance of dying, a person who is treated two hours after the injury will have a 30 percent chance of dying, and if treatment is delayed more then two hours a person with this injury will more likely die than survive. Although the time factor varies with the patient, its importance has been established beyond doubt by the experience of emergency medical technicians, traumatologists, and emergency physicians.

In the field, trauma arrest following blunt injury is virtually 100 percent fatal. Therefore, the overriding consideration of the emergency medical technician is to prevent trauma arrest in the field. The best way to do this is to decrease the period at risk—that is, the time spent in the field—and to provide the highest *quality of trauma care*, which is the last trauma-outcome determinant. Quality of trauma care must be applied across the entire continuum of trauma management, from early notification, prompt dispatch, skilled extrication and field resuscitation, clear communication, and orderly transport to the appropriate facility, to immediate and competent emergency and surgical treatment, and finally to quality intensive-care, and rehabilitative support in the hospital.

This book focuses on the last trauma-outcome determinant—the quality of trauma care—in the prehospital setting. Because of the critical importance of the time factor, decisions regarding each resuscitative step, each assessment parameter, each stabilization technique, the appropriate form of transport, and the selection of the receiving facility must all be made in the context of a time–benefit ratio. These decisions require judgment, and good judgment requires experience.

Emergency medical technicians shoulder a heavy responsibility in making decisions that can mean the difference between life and death, or between full recovery and long-term impairment. But despite their best efforts at medical control and observation of field protocol, they will always encounter pitfalls. We have therefore provided "Caution Boxes" throughout the text citing the hazards of specific injuries to both patient and health care provider, the possible dangers of decisions to utilize or omit certain techniques, and so on. These cautions serve to remind us that emergency trauma care, though a humanitarian endeavor of high calling, is not without risk.

Trauma Update for the Emergency Medical Technician is dedicated to the thousands of emergency medical technicians—the unsung heroes in the never-ending battle to reduce the mortality and morbidity of the disease known as trauma.

ACKNOWLEDGMENTS

The secretarial assistance and perseverance of Suzanne G. Lewis is gratefully acknowledged.

Kimball I. Maull
Jackie Kirby
Dennis Rowe

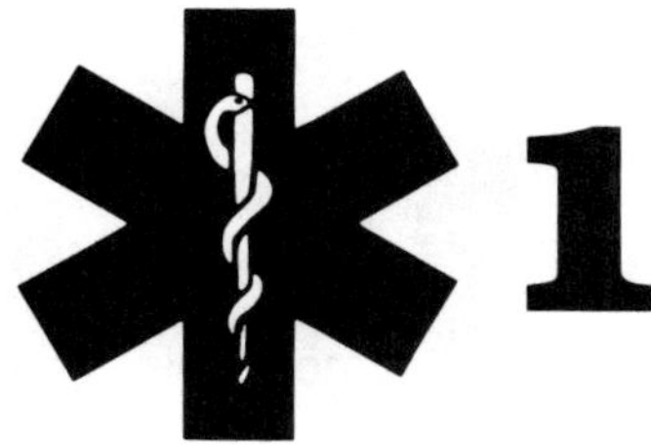

1

Kinematics

INTRODUCTION

In the field, the EMT is the eyes and ears and hands of the physician. The EMT's observations in the field help the doctor in the hospital draw conclusions regarding the patient's need for treatment and its urgency. Most physicians have little or no experience with scene work. The EMT does. Therefore, it is important for the EMT not only to observe scene findings calling attention to patterns of injury, but also to draw certain conclusions. Often, scene findings and clinical findings are closely related. For example, a collapsed steering wheel indicates a major force applied to the chest. A collapsed steering wheel is a scene finding; a fractured sternum is a clinical finding. Together, they indicate cause and effect. The EMT must communicate scene findings, even if only suspicious rather than conclusive, to hospital personnel. Omissions may lead to delay in diagnosis and treatment.

Caution!
You are the link between the trauma scene and hospital care. What is obvious to you in the field may be missed in the emergency unit—communicate!

OBJECTIVES

At the conclusion of this chapter, you should be able to:

1. Define kinematics and its significance in the management of injured patients.
2. Describe the significant differences between blunt and penetrating trauma.
3. Define the *three-level injury syndrome* of the unrestrained driver and how it relates to apparent and inapparent injuries.
4. Explain primary, secondary and tertiary collisions and relate them to the effects of mass and velocity.
5. Distinguish by pattern of injury the likely findings in side-impact, rear-impact, and rollover crashes.
6. Relate the protective and the potentially harmful effects of restraint systems and describe how scene findings can indicate specific injuries resulting from improper use.
7. Determine the mechanism of injury in vehicle versus pedestrian crashes, based on vehicle configuration and victim size.
8. Describe the basic wounding forces involved in penetrating trauma.

In most situations the experienced EMT can predict the victim's injuries with astonishing accuracy. This predictive ability is based on the EMT's recognition of forces of injury. The general objective of this chapter is to explore the patterns of injuries that are unique to specific situations.

KINEMATICS

Kinematics is the process of examining the trauma scene and determining what injuries may have resulted from the motion and forces involved. Basic to the concept of kinematics is kinetic energy, or the dynamic energy that is transferred from the moving object, such as a car or bullet, to the victim. The greater the kinetic energy involved in a traumatic event, the greater the chance of severe injury.

The equation for calculating kinetic energy is:

$$\text{Kinetic Energy} = \frac{M \times V^2}{2}$$

In the case of a motor vehicle crash, *M* represents the mass, or weight, of the patient. *V* represents the velocity, or speed, that the victim was traveling at the time of injury. V^2 means that the velocity is squared, or multiplied by itself. For example, if a car was traveling at 60 mph, V^2 would equal 3600 (60×60). The values of *M* and V^2 are multiplied, and the result is divided by 2.

The EMT is not expected to calculate the kinetic energy at the injury scene. However he or she *is* expected to understand that the more significant determinant of kinetic energy is *V*, the speed. To illustrate this, let us examine two car crashes. In both situations the driver, a 175-pound man, hits a tree. In the first crash, he was traveling at 35 mph. In the second, he was traveling twice as fast—70 mph.

Example 1

$$\text{Kinetic Energy} = 175 \times (35 \times 35) = \frac{214{,}375}{2} = 107{,}187$$

Example 2

$$\text{Kinetic Energy} = 175 \times (70 \times 70) = \frac{857{,}500}{2} = 428{,}750$$

Because the speed is squared (V^2), variations in speed can greatly affect kinetic energy. In the examples just presented, the kinetic energy quadrupled whereas the speed only doubled.

BLUNT TRAUMA

Blunt trauma refers to injuries caused by nonpenetrating forces. Common causes of blunt trauma include motor vehicle and bicycle crashes; pedestrian injuries; falls; explosions; and certain types of industrial and farm mishaps. Although penetration of the body surface may be evident following blunt trauma, and although blunt and penetrating trauma can occur together, blunt trauma usually results in internal injuries. Blunt trauma is usually caused by forces of deceleration (sudden stopping), forces of acceleration (sudden moving), or crushing forces (sudden compression).

Motor Vehicle Crashes

Motor vehicle crashes kill 50,000 Americans each year—more than the number of Americans killed during the 13-year Vietnam War. If an individual lives to be 75, his or her lifetime odds of being severely injured in a car crash are 1 in 2; of being killed, 1 in 50. Car crashes kill more Americans between the ages of 1 and 34 than any other cause. Seventy percent of deaths and injuries occur at speeds of 40 mph or less and no more than five miles from home.

Patterns of injury in car crashes are often predictable, but a number of variables can affect injury severity. These variables include:

1. force and direction of the collision;
2. shape and texture of the opposing surface;
3. energy-absorbing characteristics of the opposing object; and
4. restraints.

A head-on collision will produce a different set of injuries than a rear-end collision. A high-speed crash is more lethal than a fender-bender. A person who hits a rigid steering wheel will be injured differently from a person who hits a padded dashboard. Finally, a restrained occupant is typically injured less severely than an unrestrained rider. Once the EMT knows the direction of the impact, the speed involved, whether or not restraints were used, and the victim's position in the car, he or she can predict the pattern of injuries. This predictive ability contributes immeasurably to the prehospital care the victim receives.

One Crash, Three Collisions. Suppose a car traveling at 55 mph strikes a tree head-on. Three collisions actually occur in such a crash. First, the car hits the solid object and abruptly stops. But the occupant continues to travel forward at 55 mph. The second collision occurs when the unrestrained occupant's body hits the interior of the car and stops. However, the victim's heart, liver, brain, and other organs continue forward at 55 mph, until they hit the internal structures of the body—the third collision. Each collision can cause damage, and each consumes a portion of the kinetic energy released in the crash.

Head-On Impact. Approximately 50 percent of motor vehicle deaths occur in head-on crashes. The three collisions just described occur in less than one second. Even if the occupant anticipates the impact, the forces are so great that it is impossible to adequately brace oneself to prevent injury.

Injuries to the unrestrained driver commonly occur together at three distinct levels:

level 1: head and neck, including facial injury

level 2: chest and abdomen

level 3: lower extremity and pelvis

This *three-level injury syndrome* of the unrestrained driver has clinical significance because head (especially face) and lower-extremity injuries are usually obvious. Coupled with scene evidence, the EMT should suspect internal injuries to the chest and abdomen (Figure 1.1). Almost any injury or combination of injuries can occur when the patient is ejected from the vehicle.

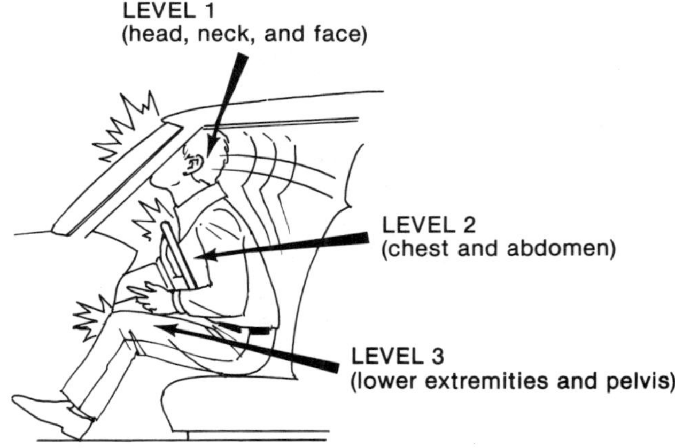

FIGURE 1.1 The three-level injury syndrome of the unrestrained driver.

When the front of the car hits a solid object and stops, the unrestrained occupant will continue to move forward at the same speed as the car. In a 30 mph crash, the knees hit the instrument panel .006 seconds after the car hits the object. The force of impact is transmitted to the upper leg. A fractured femur, dislocated hip, or dislocated knee may result. One one-hundredth of a second later the chest hits the steering wheel. The frequently seen bruised sternum is an excellent indication of a high-impact head-on collision. The sternum and ribs may fracture from the direct force. A fractured rib, now capable of acting as a sharp spear, may puncture the lung and cause a pneumothorax or lacerate a vessel and cause a hemothorax.

After the thorax stops its forward motion, the heart and lungs will continue to move forward until they strike the sternum and ribs. This collision can cause cardiac and pulmonary contusions—both very common in head-on crashes. If the impact occurs when the heart is in diastole (the phase when the heart is filling with blood), the force can cause the heart to rupture.

Injury to the aorta is less common, but frequently fatal. As the aorta exits the heart, it curves backward and travels down. When the heart is propelled forward in a head-on crash, the aorta is stretched and a tear can occur, usually at the origin of the left subclavian artery. If the laceration is large, the victim may bleed to death in a few seconds (Figure 1.2).

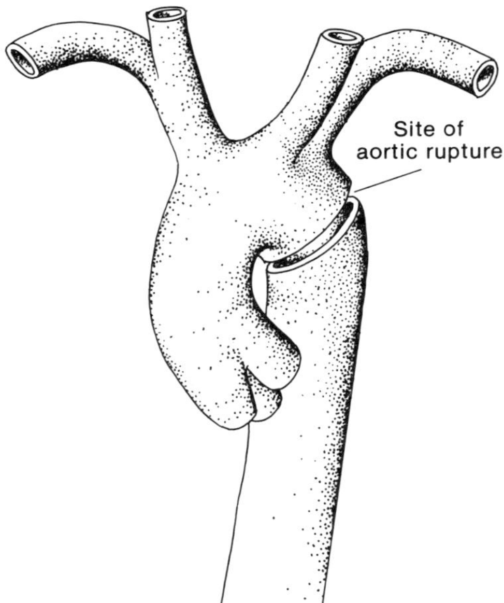

FIGURE 1.2 Most common site of aortic rupture following sudden deceleration.

A spontaneous pneumothorax can occur without any obvious cause. When this happens, it is typically because the driver anticipates the crash, takes a deep breath, and holds it. As the driver hits the steering wheel, the impact compresses the chest, but the air cannot escape because the glottis is closed. As a result, the lung ruptures, then collapses.

The victim's abdomen also hits the steering wheel. The force can increase the pressure in the abdomen and rupture the diaphragm. The tear occurs most frequently on the left side, which is unprotected by the liver, but it can occur on the right. If the tear is large enough the abdominal organs can be forced into the chest, compressing the lungs and interfering with ventilation (Figure 1.3).

Impact with the steering wheel can also injure the liver and spleen. The liver, located in the right upper abdomen, is only partially protected by the ribs. For this reason it is the most frequently injured abdominal organ. Injury to the spleen, located on the opposite side of the abdomen, is common, and delay in treatment is a major cause of preventable death.

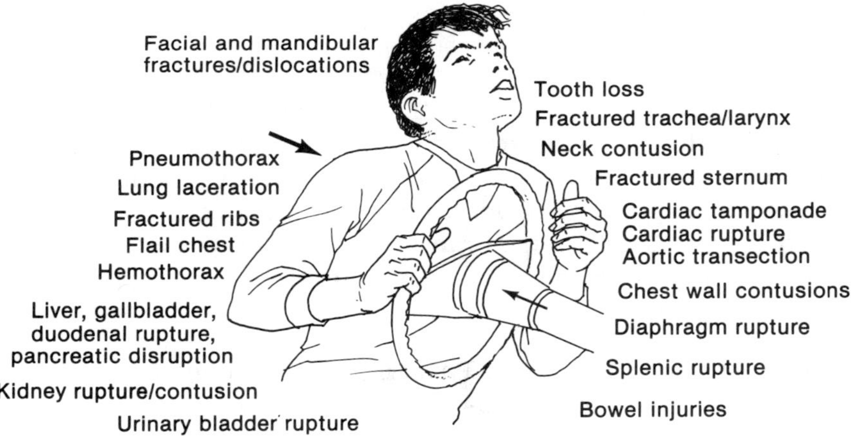

FIGURE 1.3 Level 2 injuries resulting from impact with the steering wheel.

The third and final phase of a head-on collision occurs when the head hits the windshield or car roof. In a 30 mph crash the head will bulge a laminated windshield five inches. Facial lacerations are caused by the head returning through the broken windshield. Skull fractures and head injuries are frequent. After the head hits the windshield or car roof and stops, the brain continues to move forward, hitting the inside of the skull and possibly sustaining a cerebral contusion. Also, the interior of the skull has irregular protrusions that can lacerate the brain as it moves forward. Finally, the violent forward motion can cause the meninges to pull away from the skull, causing ruptured blood vessels and cerebral hemorrhage. (Figure 1.4).

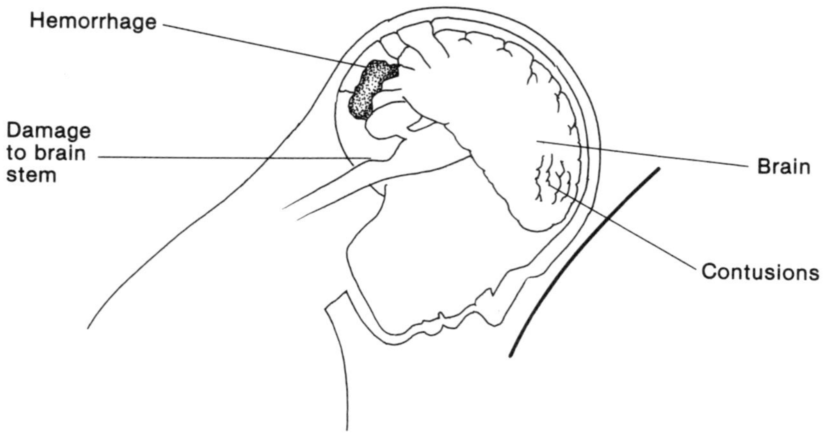

FIGURE 1.4 Level 1 injuries to the head, face, and neck resulting from impact with the windshield or car roof.

As the head whips forward, the cervical spine can either flex or extend. If the neck is flexed forward and rotated, the impact can cause unstable and potentially paralyzing fractures or dislocations of the cervical spine. If impact occurs with the neck extended and rotated, a C2 or (hangman's) fracture can result. Cervical spine injuries, even unstable ones, may not be immediately apparent, but must be suspected in all deceleration incidents.

Unrestrained Back-seat Passengers. In a head-on collision, the unrestrained back-seat passenger moves forward, hits the rear of the front seat, and may somersault into the front seat (Figure 1.5). The unrestrained back-seat passenger may cause significant rear-loading injuries to the restrained front-seat passenger and is therefore a real threat.

Side Impact. Side impact collisions occur in 20 percent of all car crashes, and is one of the most dangerous. If the car occupant is hit by another car, the force is delivered below the neck. If the collision involves a higher vehicle, such as a truck, the head is affected.

Typically, such a collision forces the occupant's body out from under the head , causing cervical fractures. Direct force can also fracture the clavicle, ribs, femur, and pelvis. If the driver is hit, spleen injuries are common. If someone on the passenger's side is hit, liver injuries are likely (Figure 1.6).

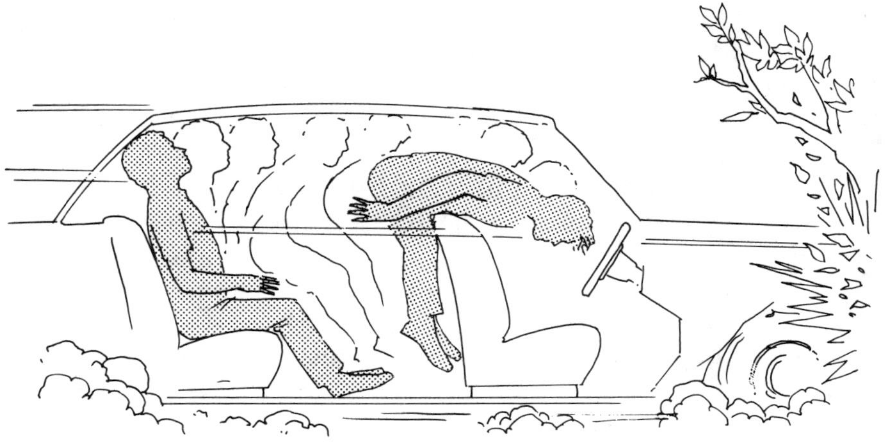

FIGURE 1.5 The "second collision" of the unrestrained rear passenger.

Safety belts cannot prevent direct injuries in this type of crash. But they can prevent ejection, protect the opposite passenger, and prevent occupants from being flung across the car and striking the opposite side. Also, a restrained driver is more capable of retaining control of the motor vehicle and avoiding secondary collisions.

Rear-End Impact. In a rear-end collision, the car is hit from behind and propelled forward. The occupant's body is pushed out

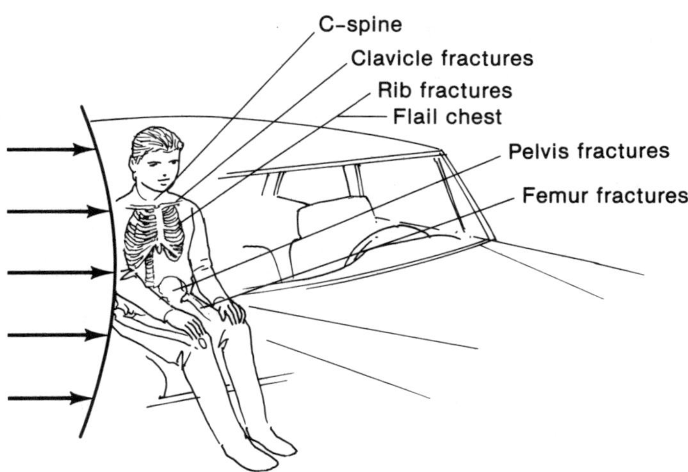

FIGURE 1.6 Result of vehicle intrusion in a side-impact collision.

from under the neck and head. The head is whipped backwards, then forward—hence the term *whiplash* (Figure 1.7). Whiplash causes violent stretching and tearing of the muscles and ligaments. Symptoms are usually progressive and often prolonged and painful.

Ninety percent of whiplash injuries occur when the victim is sitting in a stationary car and is hit from the rear at an average speed of only 15 mph. The majority of whiplash cases could be prevented if headrests were properly adjusted (Figure 1.8).

If the car that is hit rolls forward gently before coming to rest, injuries are usually limited. However, the vehicle is often pushed into another object or into the path of an oncoming vehicle, resulting in a second collision; multiple energy transfers occur, and injuries may be less predictable.

Roll-over Crashes. The roll-over crash, though often spectacular, produces less severe injuries than other types of crashes, provided the occupants are restrained and not ejected. The kinetic energy is dissipated in small amounts over a large distance. Because of the complex distribution of forces, specific injuries are less predictable in roll-over crashes than in other types of crashes.

Ejection. If the victim is ejected from the vehicle, the extent and severity of the injuries increase dramatically. Partial ejection typically results in crush and avulsion injuries. Total ejection accounts for 27 percent of all trauma deaths. It is associated with a 300 percent increase in mortality and a 1,300 percent increase in the incidence of cervical spine injuries. Disfiguring soft-tissue trauma is common in victims of ejection.

Caution!
If the victim is ejected, injury patterns cannot be predicted with accuracy and the injury is usually more severe.

Restraints. Safety belts are designed to absorb the kinetic energy transmitted from the car to the body and spread it out over a wide area. Properly worn, a three-point restraint, which consists of a shoulder and lap belt, dissipates the energy over the parts of the body having the highest tolerance levels—the pelvis and upper torso. Restraints secure the body to the frame of the car, preventing ejection and limiting contact between the occupant and the car interior.

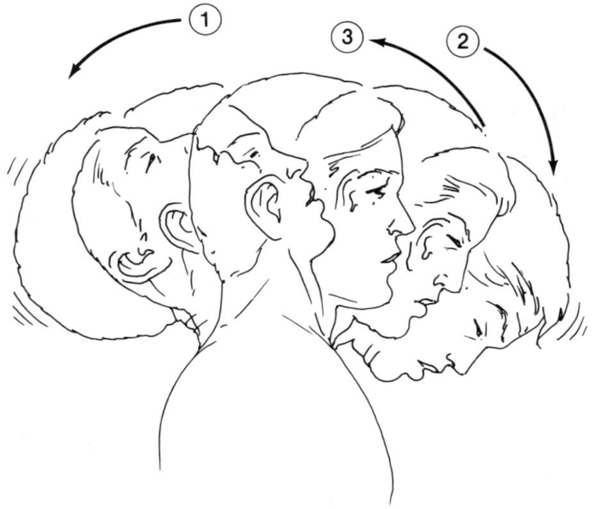

FIGURE 1.7 Head and neck motion resulting from sudden rear loading.

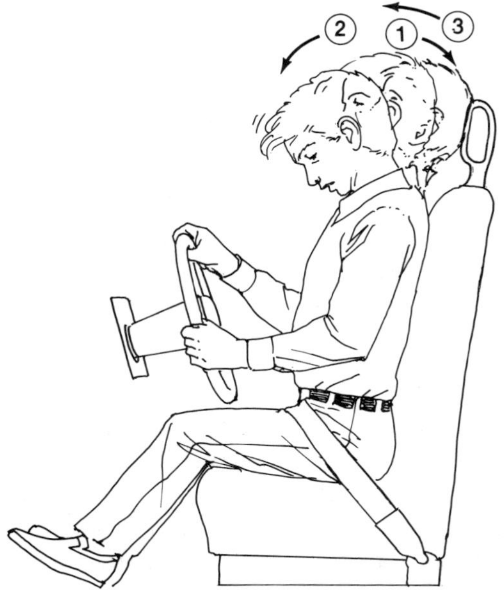

FIGURE 1.8 Protective effect of properly adjusted heardrest.

Although the use of safety belts dramatically reduces the incidence and severity of injury, improper use can lead to specific injuries (Figure 1.9). These injuries are especially apparent in head-on crashes where the victim has a loosely fitting lap belt worn over the mid-abdomen instead of across the iliac crest. In a crash, the victim is propelled forward, flexing around the lap belt. The resulting compression can injure the lower spinal cord and the abdominal organs, such as the liver, spleen, and small bowel, as well as increasing intro-adbominal pressure and rupturing the diaphragm.

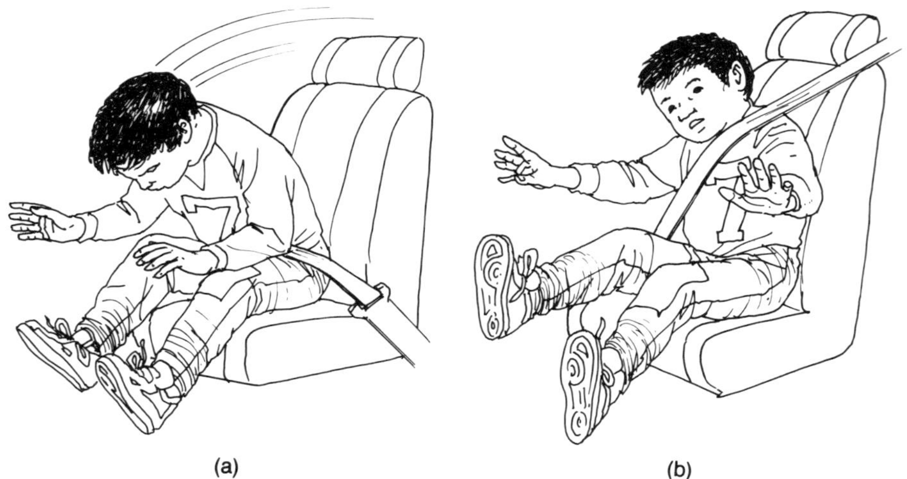

(a) (b)

FIGURE 1.9 Problems resulting from improper safety belt use: (a) high riding lap belt compresses abdomen and lumbar spine (b) diagonal belt alone jeopardizes head, neck, and lower torso.

> **Caution!**
> Improperly worn safety restraints are dangerous—note whether belts were used and, if so, whether they were applied properly.

All automobiles manufactured after 1989 must be equipped with air bags or passive restraint systems. The latter though, may be simply a diagonal strap that automatically restrains the front-seat occupants. This system is designed so that the occupant must *actively* fasten the lap belt to be properly restrained. If the occupant does not fasten the lap belt and the car is involved in a head-on collision, severe injuries can occur. As the occupant is propelled forward, the unrestrained lower torso can move down and under the steering wheel. The occupant's chin can catch on the diagonal strap, causing severe neck injuries and even decapitation.

Pedestrian–Motor Vehicle Crashes

Injury patterns associated with car–pedestrian crashes depend upon the height of the victim and the type of vehicle. An adult typically turns away from an oncoming car. The car bumper may strike the knees and the hood may hit the pelvis, causing extensive open and/or closed fractures of the lower extremities. The victim is then thrown onto the hood of the car, and when the driver slams on the brakes, the victim slides off the hood and hits the road.

Because a child is smaller, a different injury pattern is seen. The child often turns to face the car. The bumper typically hits the child's femur and pelvis, and the hood hits the chest. Since his center of gravity is lower, the child may be thrown forward and land on his head. The child is then in danger of being run over by the same car, or landing in the path of an oncoming vehicle. Because the pedestrian is unprotected, the injuries are often fatal.

Falls

All falls are potentially serious, especially in the elderly. Regardless of age, falls from more than three times one's height can cause major trauma. If the victim lands on the feet, the calcaneus (heel bone) is frequently fractured. The energy from the fall is then transmitted to the lumbar and thoracic spine, causing compression fractures and spinal cord injuries (Figure 1.10). The victim may fall forward and sustain wrist fractures as she tries to protect herself from the fall (Figure 1.11).

If the individual stumbles and falls forward, the energy is distributed over the ankle, knee, wrist, shoulder, and face. Although this type of fall may cause only minor injuries in children and adults, it can cause multiple fractures in the elderly, whose bones are weakened by osteoporosis.

Landing in a sitting position typically causes thoracic spine and cord injuries. This injury is frequently seen in survivors of plane crashes.

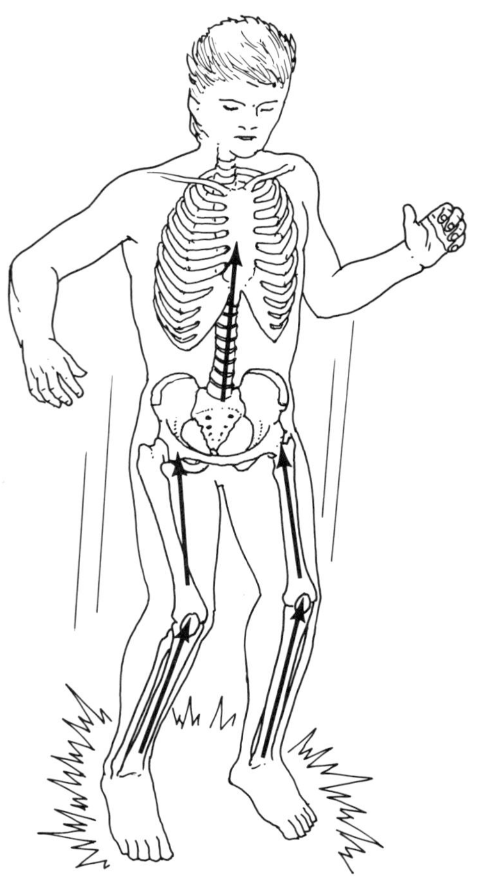

FIGURE 1.10 Transmission of forces in vertical-deceleration injury.

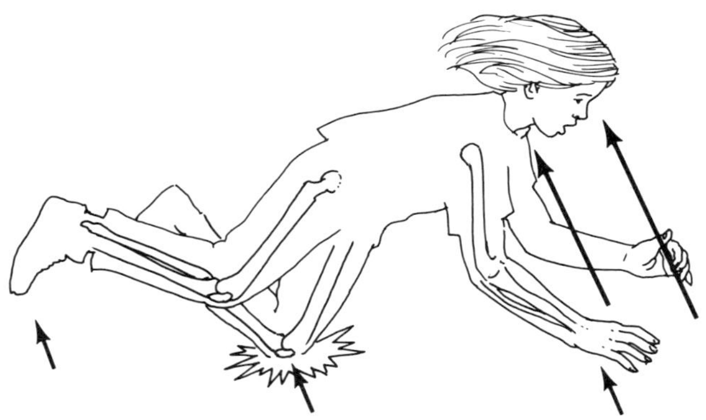

FIGURE 1.11 Falling forward results in a wider distribution of forces.

PENETRATING TRAUMA

Injuries associated with penetrating trauma can be classified according to the kinetic energy, which in this case is a product of missile size and speed. The kinetic energy can be low, very high, or any point in between.

Low-Energy Penetrating Trauma. This includes injuries caused by knives, ice picks, and bullets fired from handguns. Tissue damage is limited to the tract between the entrance and exit. If there is no exit wound, field estimation of the extent of injury may not be possible. Unless a low-energy missile hits a vital organ, such as the heart, aorta, or brain, the injury is usually survivable if promptly recognized and properly treated.

High-Energy Penetrating Trauma. This is caused by missiles fired from powerful rifles such as hunting weapons. The missile strikes the tissue with great velocity, causing massive destruction (Figure 1.12). The tissue damage is proportional to the kinetic energy of the bullet as it enters the body, minus the energy that remains as it exits. Unfortunately, many modern bullets are designed to flatten, fragment, and tumble upon impact. This design slows the bullet's passage through the tissue, and more tissue-damaging kinetic energy can thereby be released.

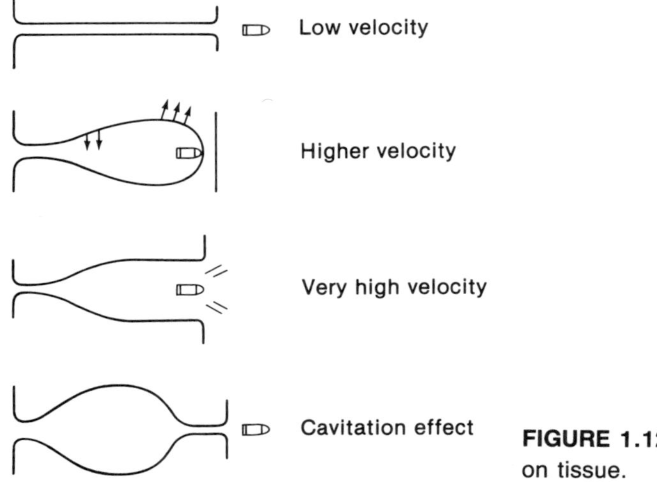

FIGURE 1.12 Effects of a missile on tissue.

Another damaging effect of high-velocity missiles is cavitation. As the bullet passes through tissue, it transmits explosive energy to the tissue much like a shock wave. A huge cavity, much larger than the size of the bullet, is created by these waves. The tissue recoils, only to spring back. The higher the density of the tissue, the greater the damage from cavitation. For example, the liver receives severe cavitation, the lungs much less.

Caution!
Internal injury resulting from high-velocity missiles may occur beyond the obvious missile tract.

CONCLUSION

Kinematics involves detecting the mechanism of injury—an invaluable source of information in diagnosing the site and severity of the injury. As an EMT, you will often have firsthand knowledge of the mechanism of injury. Be observant and communicate what you see to those responsible for patient care. A wise clinician will listen.

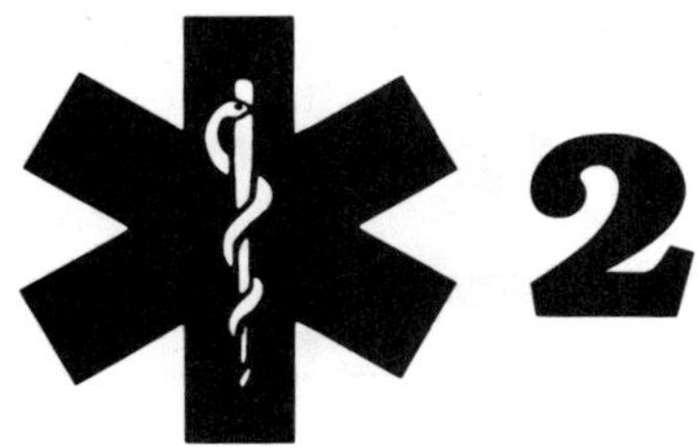

2

Initial Evaluation

INTRODUCTION

In the early 1960s, R. Adams Cowley, director of the Shock-Trauma Center in Baltimore, Maryland, established a principle still widely accepted today —multiple trauma patients who receive definitive care within 60 minutes have greatly improved chances of recovery. He concluded that the mortality rate for multiple-trauma patients would triple for every 60 minutes beyond that "golden hour" between the incident and the provision of definitive care. When dealing with the injured, the EMT becomes the guardian of the golden hour. Every measure taken in the field takes time, whether it is an assessment function or an intervention. The EMT must be mindful of the risk–benefit ratio of everything done. Delay in provision of definitive care is the ever-present risk for the patient and a source of stress for the EMT. Field trauma care can best be expedited by a logical, well-defined, and practical plan of trauma assessment and management. It is the purpose of this chapter to outline such an approach.

Saving time for the trauma patient begins prior to dispatch and must be considered in forming a plan of action. The aid vehicle must be thoroughly supplied and equipped, and all items must be in working order. Thorough knowledge of the geographic area is essential; the EMT should know the shortest route (1) to the scene and (2) from the scene to the appropriate definitive-care facility. Emergency care crews should be familiar with area maps and know where they are kept in the vehicle.

When dispatched, the EMT should write down the information immediately and accurately. An incorrect location or poor directions increase response time and cause unnecessary delay.

Caution!
Trauma arrest in the field is uniformly fatal. All efforts at assessment and treatment should be directed at saving time and preventing field trauma arrest.

OBJECTIVES

At the completion of this chapter, you should be able to:

1. Develop a plan of action in approaching a scene where there are one or more trauma victims.
2. Categorize trauma patients according to the urgency of their need for treatment.
3. Define stability and describe how it is used and misused in prehospital and interhospital communication.
4. Demonstrate priorities in patient assessment and management.
5. Explain secondary survey in trauma rescue, and describe risk-benefit ratio in field assessment and intervention.
6. Explain why certain patients are at greater risk for no apparent cervical spine injury and why virtually all victims of blunt trauma require c-spine immobilization.
7. Demonstrate how to detect pelvic fracture.
8. Determine which patients require immediate transport and which do not.

PLAN OF ACTION

The following principles apply to most trauma situations. Once you reach the scene, make a quick assessment of the incident. Park as close as possible without compromising safety. Watch for hazards as you get out of your vehicle. Do not run! Walk purposefully toward the patients, being cautious and observant. Confirm the mechanism of injury—crash, shooting, fire, or whatever—and locate all victims. Perform patient triage, prioritize the patient's injuries, and stabilize and package for transport. Load the patient into the ambulance quickly but gently. Choose the hospital according to the needs of the patient. The most experienced person should stay with the patient and continuously monitor his or her status. After addressing any life-threatening conditions, contact Medical Control and relay the victim's condition, estimated arrival time, and any anticipated special needs.

Do not abandon the patient at the hospital. Continue care until relieved by emergency-department personnel. Give a complete report to the physician or nurse in charge. Complete the response form and ready the vehicle for subsequent service.

Use the CUPS system for categorizing trauma patients. This system involves four distinct condition categories:

*C*PR: The patient is in respiratory or cardiac arrest.

*U*nstable: the patient is in shock, with or without accompanying respiratory distress.

*P*otentially unstable: The patient has marginal vital signs and requires close monitoring. This victim's survivability may well be affected by transport or treatment delay.

*S*table: The patient is in no distress. Vital signs are normal and there are no respiratory problems.

Caution!
Stability implies a steady state over time. Certain patients should be regarded as potentially unstable based on the mechanism of injury, even if they show normal vital signs.

Use CUPS when trying to decide which patient should be treated and transported first. Continually reassess the patient's condition and update the CUPS category as necessary.

EARLY MANAGEMENT

Orderly trauma management should become almost automatic. Memorize the following steps and be prepared to perform them in the correct sequence:

1. Maintain an open airway and stabilize the cervical spine.
2. Determine adequacy of ventilation.
3. Control hemorrhage.
4. Treat shock.
5. Assess for other injuries, perform a brief neurological examination, and splint major fractures.
6. Transport the patient, constantly monitoring and reassessing his or her condition.

Always remember—by following this approach, you can perform a rapid primary survey, resuscitation of vital functions, and a secondary survey, all within a few minutes.

> **Caution!**
> In certain situations, you may not be able to complete the secondary assessment of your patient. Findings from the primary survey may dictate immediate transport; the secondary survey can be performed during transport or when at the hospital.

Begin your primary assessment as soon as you gain access to the patient. Patient entrapment may require you to continue assessment and early management during extrication. Approach the patient from the head and maintain cervical immobilization while determining that the patient is breathing. Assess the patient for a patent airway. Quickly check the airway for blood, foreign debris, vomitus, or any other obstruction. Evaluate the rate, frequency, depth, and pattern of ventilation. If the airway is obstructed, open it with a jaw thrust (Figure 2.1). Don't extend the neck to open the airway; to do so increases the risk of spinal cord injury. Any difficulty in breathing should be immediately treated with oxygen at high concentration. Respiratory distress should alert you to chest injuries or a deterioration of the patient's condition.

Manually stabilize the neck in neutral position, and do not release control of it until you are relieved by another trained person or until a stabilization device is applied. At this point, it is often convenient to check for carotid pulse, midline tracheal location, and spinal tenderness.

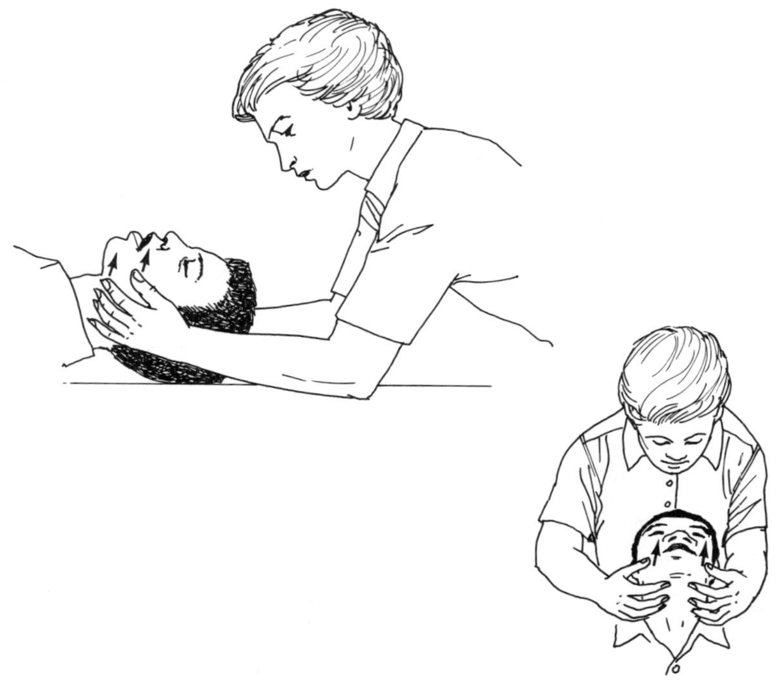

FIGURE 2.1 Jaw thrust: Open the airway by bringing the moncible forward without extending the cervical spine.

Next, examine the chest. Inspect for sucking chest wounds, flail segments, bruising, or notable deformity. Note if the chest goes in and out equally with each breath, and whether each ventilation leads to full expansion or whether it involves movement of the abdominal muscles only. The latter occurs passively with contraction of the diaphragm and indicates cervical spine injury below the C2 or C3 level. Palpate for broken ribs and subcutaneous emphysema. If breath sounds are decreased or absent on one side, percuss the chest for hyperresonant or dull sounds. Hyperresonance indicates pneumothorax; dull sounds suggest hemothorax (see Chapter 4).

External bleeding should be under control at this point. A crew member or a first-responder should control bleeding while you evaluate the airway, breathing, and circulation. Direct pressure is the best way to control bleeding (Figure 2.2). Use of tourniquets should be restricted to near amputations that are not amenable to pressure control. Air splints and pneumatic antishock garments

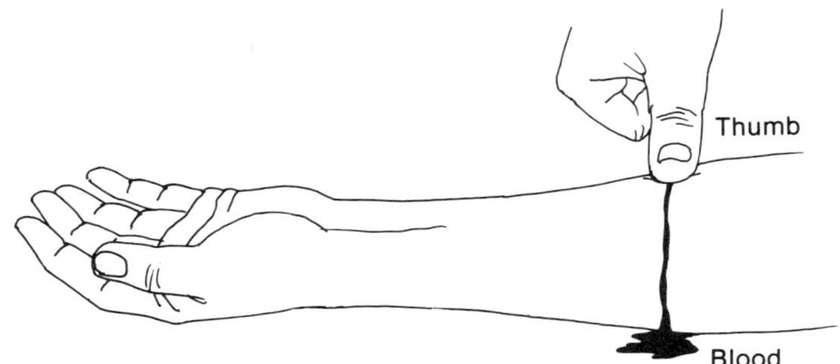

FIGURE 2.2 Your fingers are an excellent hemostatic device—use them.

may be useful to control bleeding depending on the site and extent of hemorrhage.

> **Caution!**
> Brisk internal bleeding is rapidly fatal and cannot be controlled in the field. Know your transport times.

Record the blood pressure, but remember that a fall in blood pressure is a relatively late sign of shock. A pale, cool, clammy, confused, weak, thirsty, or sweating patient is in shock regardless of blood pressure reading. The preceding signs and symptoms indicate hemorrhagic shock and may appear before the blood pressure drops. Spinal shock may occur without tachycardia, vasoconstriction, or diaphoresis.

The best treatment for shock is anticipation. Virtually all patients in shock should be provided with high-flow oxygen. Use of the pneumatic antishock garment (PASG) may be indicated. The patient should be taken to a facility that can provide immediate surgical care.

As soon as you complete these initial resuscitative efforts, begin your secondary survey. If the patient is unstable, omit or postpone this survey until transport is under way. In your secondary survey, recheck the patient from head to toe. Reassess vital signs and compare them with earlier findings.

Do a brief neurological examination. Check:

1. Level of consciousness:
   A—alert

V—responds to verbal stimuli
P—responds only to pain
U—unresponsive

2. Motor ability: Can patient move fingers and/or toes?
3. Sensation: Does patient respond to touch or pain?
4. Pupils: Are they equal or unequal, and do they react to light?

Examine the abdomen. Observe for signs of blunt or penetrating trauma, including contusion, penetrating wounds, and distention. Palpate the abdomen for tenderness. If the abdomen is distended, tender, or rigid, assume that the victim is bleeding internally. Do not waste time listening for bowel sounds.

Quickly check the pelvis for tenderness or instability (Figure 2.3). Massive blood loss can occur from pelvic fractures, and improper handling may aggravate the bleeding. Minimize moving the pelvis if you suspect major blunt pelvic trauma.

At this point, splint fractures and check distal sensation and pulses on all extremities. Be sure to check again after straightening any fractures. Splint fractures according to your local training.

Injuries above the clavicles including maxillofacial trauma, place the patient at higher risk for associated cervical spine injuries. In such a case, ensure complete cervical spine immobilization before transport. Patients without evidence of trauma above the clavicles may also have cervical spine injury. It is easy to be fooled. Pedestrian–vehicle crashes, rear-end collisions, and improper safety belt use are all potential settings for cervical spine injury. Perhaps the greatest pitfall in your secondary survey is that an awake patient may have other painful injuries that distract you. This patient typically does not complain of neck pain yet may have an unstable neck injury.

Obtain as much history of the injury as possible, including the mechanism of injury, state of consciousness, use of restraints, and damage to the vehicle. Check also for a Medic Alert tag.

Contact Medical Control as needed to secure management directions and to report the patient's condition. The more critical the patient's condition, the sooner you should contact Medical Control and transport the patient.

When reporting to Medical Control, use the following guidelines:

1. Identify yourself; give your level of training and your organization.

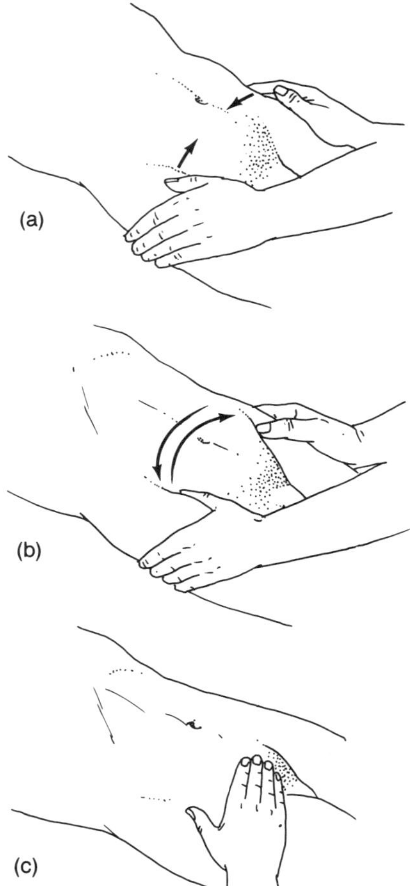

FIGURE 2.3 Compression–distraction maneuver for checking pelvic stability. Free movement or crepitus (grating) suggests a fracture.

2. Give the patient's age, sex, injuries, vital signs, state of consciousness, and condition category (CUPS).
3. Perform life-support procedures endorsed by your EMS and consistent with your level of training.
4. Transport the patient to the facility best able to deliver trauma care for your area, or as directed by Medical Control.
5. Notify the facility of the estimated time of arrival, and the condition of the patient, and ask for orders needed for additional management of the patient. Report any special support that will be needed upon arrival.

Minutes are important to the trauma patient—if you are not helping, you best be moving! Constantly monitor and reevaluate the patient during transport. Notify Medical Control if the patient's condition deteriorates. Record all that you see and do, including times, circumstances, and significant details.

> **Caution!**
> Stabilization in the field can be fatal to the critically injured patient.

LOAD-AND-GO SITUATIONS

Certain injuries demand immediate transport of the patient. Load the patient immediately onto a backboard and transport rapidly to the closest appropriate trauma facility. Perform lifesaving procedures along the way. Basic Trauma Life Support (BTLS) recognizes the following as load-and-go situations:

1. airway obstruction that cannot be quickly relieved by mechanical methods such as suction or position
2. trauma-induced cardiorespiratory arrest
3. tension pneumothorax
4. pericardial tamponade
5. penetrating wounds of the chest accompanied by shock
6. massive hemothorax accompanied by shock
7. head injury with rapidly deteriorating neurologic status or unilaterally dilated pupil

> **Caution!**
> Lives saved in the field can be lost in the emergency unit. Make sure the patient is transported to a facility that can provide immediate definitive care.

CONCLUSION

Your initial assessment of the victim is often the most important assessment that he or she receives. It identifies conditions that are immediately life-threatening and prioritizes the patient's management. The first rule of trauma care is to do no further harm. For many patients, delay is harmful. Thus, you must perform your initial assessment quickly but accurately.

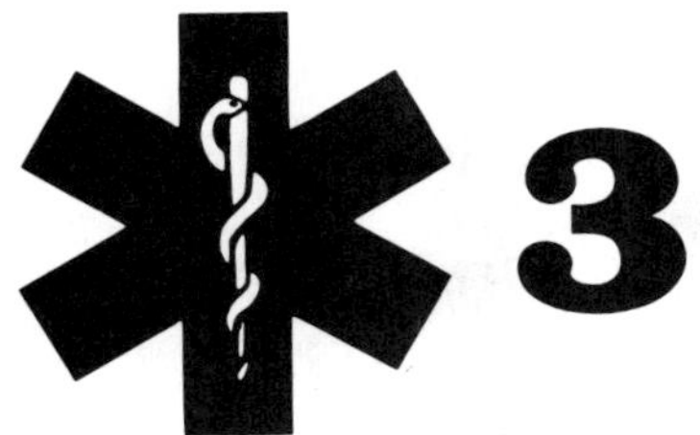

3

Upper Airway Management and Ventilation

INTRODUCTION

Maintaining an open airway and adequate ventilation has priority over every other emergency technique, whether the patient has a heart attack, a gunshot wound, or a traffic mishap. The rule is always the same—the airway and breathing come first. Circulation of unoxygenated blood is of no use to the body; its organs will soon die without *immediate* and *decisive* action. Even partial blockage of the airway and ventilation can lead to critical complications for the patient. Airway care is especially challenging since it includes the added responsibilities of maintaining neck and spine immobilization and treating the patient's injuries while dealing with the difficult complications often found in the field.

In this chapter we examine airway care and ventilation of injured patients. We will review the basic structure of the upper airway, ways it may be compromised, and recognition and treatment of upper airway crisis. We will also describe manual and mechanical methods of airway care and ventilation.

OBJECTIVES

At the completion of this chapter, you will be able to:

1. Describe the components of the upper airway, their location, their function, and the basic physiology of breathing.
2. Explain the importance of the airway and breathing and their priority in trauma care.
3. Describe the signs and symptoms of a comprised airway in the trauma victim.
4. Give examples of the various methods (both manual and mechanical) of maintaining the airway and ventilation without injuring the cervical spine.
5. Distinguish the use, maintenance, and limitations of mechanical aids to the airway and ventilation.

ANATOMY AND PHYSIOLOGY OF THE UPPER AIRWAY

The airway is divided into upper and lower sections by the vocal cords (larynx). The upper airway (Figure 3.1) consists of:

The *oral cavity* (mouth), which includes the tongue, teeth, and gums.

The *nasal passages.* These are not usually of critical importance unless the oral air passage is blocked or heavy bleeding from the nasal cavity compromises the airway. Keep in mind that infants do not breathe through their mouths until they are about six months old. Occlusion of their nasal passages is therefore critical.

The *pharynx* (throat).

The *epiglottis*—a flaplike valve that closes upon swallowing to prevent food and other materials from entering the trachea.

The *larynx*—The Adam's Apple or voice box which contains the vocal cords.

Below the larynx is the *lower* airway (Figure 3.2), which consists of:

The *trachea* (windpipe)—divides at the carina into bronchial tubes.

The *bronchial tubes*—the two divisions of the trachea, one going to each lung.

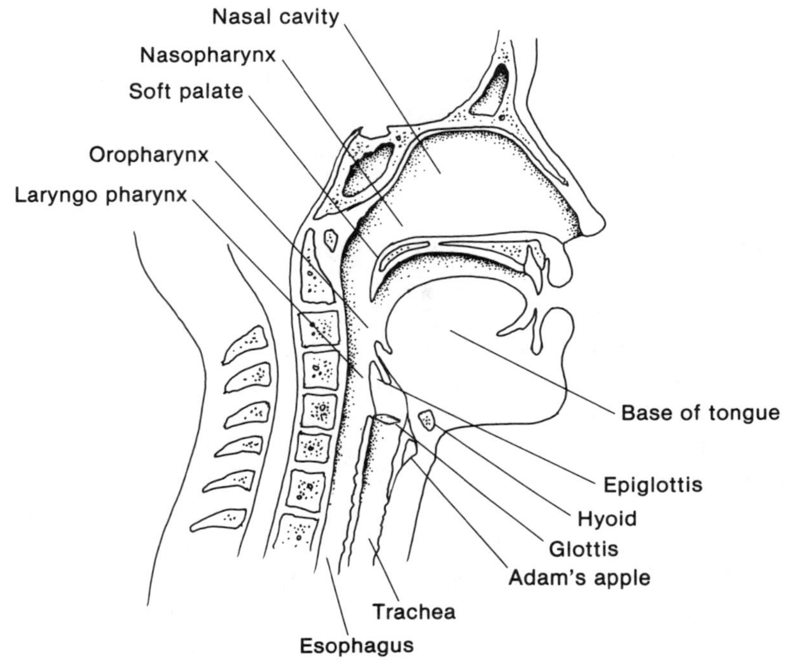

FIGURE 3.1 Anatomy of upper airway.

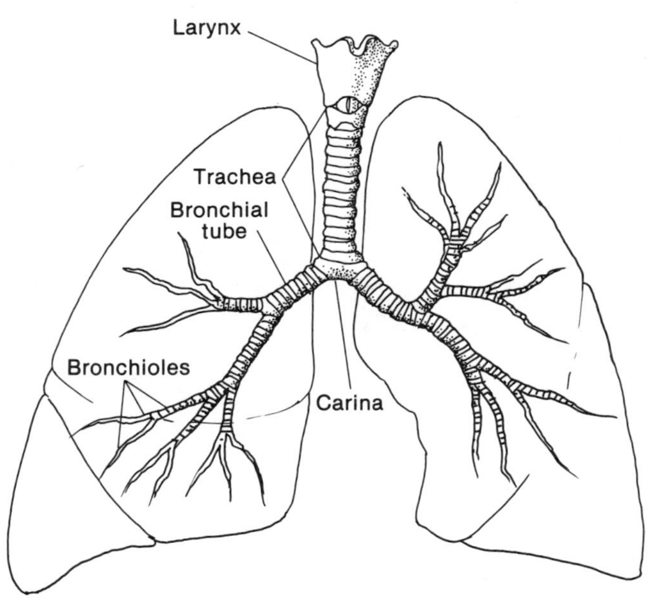

FIGURE 3.2 Anatomy of lower airway.

The *bronchioles*—The small, treelike divisions of the bronchial tubes.

The *alveoli*—the tiny, elastic air sac where oxygen and carbon dioxide are exchanged.

In this chapter we are principally concerned with problems of the *upper* airway. It is important, however, to familiarize yourself with the overall respiratory process to fully appreciate the importance of the upper airway and ventilation.

Upon inspiration (inhalation), the chest cavity enlarges due to expansion of the chest wall muscles and flattening of the diaphragm (Figure 3.3). As a result, the air pressure inside the chest drops below the atmospheric pressure outside the body, creating a vacuum. "Nature abhors a vacuum" and will try to fill it (in this case the lungs) by using the path of least resistance (the airways). This is the process of inspiration. The process is then reversed: The chest wall and diaphragm contract, shrinking the chest cavity, increasing internal pressure, and forcing the air in the lungs out—exhalation. This simplified version of respiration clearly shows the importance of an unobstructed airway for ventilation and oxygenation. For a more detailed explanation, consult the discussion of chest anatomy and physiology in Chapter 4.

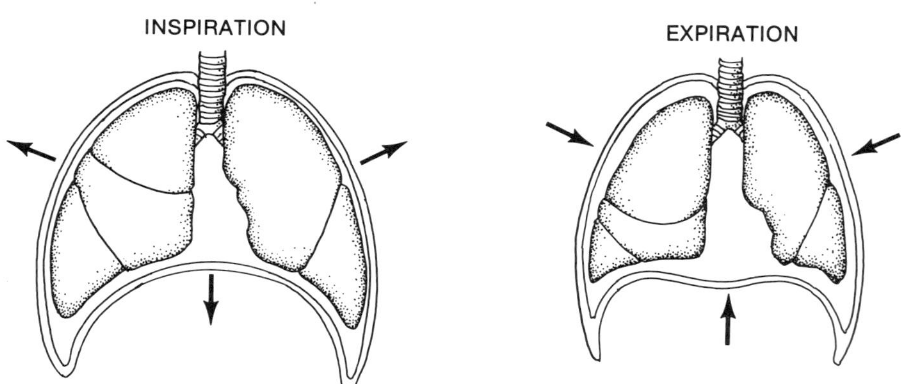

FIGURE 3.3 Normal inspiration and expiration.

KEEPING THE AIRWAY OPEN

Even if patients have no airway blockage, you must make sure the airway stays open. You can do this through preventive airway care.

If respiration is adequate and the patient appears to be oxygenated, make sure that the airway remains patent. If the patient is alert and conscious, you must *continuously observe* his or her overall condition. Any change in condition justifies a complete reevaluation, starting, of course, with the airway and breathing. The earliest symptom of respiratory distress and hypoxia (systemic lack of oxygen) may be very subtle changes in the patient's mental state.

Even if the patient is apparently stable, you must immobilize him or her to allow airway care without spinal compromise. Fully immobilize the patient according to local protocol; this will allow safe turning should vomiting occur. Check the position of the trachea before applying a cervical collar.

THE COMPROMISED AIRWAY

Anytime the airway is blocked, respiration is endangered. Always suspect the worst, and look for subtle signs of airway and breathing problems. Certainly a blow, stab, or gunshot to the neck or face may obstruct the upper airway, and the tongue, foreign bodies, food, or vomitus may create problems just as in the nontrauma patient. Bleeding and impaled objects are also potential threats. Be ever alert for the patient who says, "I can't breathe." Often such a patient doesn't look *that* bad at the time, and associated symptoms of anxiety, restlessness, or combativeness may be misinterpreted as the result of intoxication or hysteria. If the patient tells you he can't breathe, *listen and act*! Patients become extremely anxious and agitated as they struggle to breathe.

Physical Findings

Closely evaluate the scene for possible causes of airway compromise. Look for evidence of eating, broken dentures, vomitus, or impact of the face against an object. Look for wounds, hematoma, swelling or any other deformity that would indicate direct injury. Also palpate for tracheal deviation at the suprasternal notch, which could indicate a tension pneumothorax.

Consider the patient's overall appearance. Patient's with airway blockage show varying degrees of distress; critical patients are apprehensive, struggle to breathe, and show poor color. Flaring of the nostrils may occur in persons struggling to breathe.

Intercostal retraction—retraction of the skin between the ribs during inspiration—is an important finding, as is, *suprasternal retraction,* seen just over the sternal notch. Both conditions are caused by use of the auxiliary muscles (intercostal and sternal) to improve respiration. In trying to breathe, the patient may struggle to sit up or constantly change position. Watch for change in level of consciousness. As hypoxia increases, consciousness may decrease.

Cyanosis—a bluish color that usually begins in the ear lobes, lips, and nail beds—suggests significant obstruction. Obstruction of the upper airway may be indicated by crowing or gurgling. You may hear *stridor*—a high-pitched sound in the throat caused by a partially occluded upper airway. Or you may hear *rafles* and *rhonchi* during chest auscultation; these vary from fine crackling noises to continuous gurgling. These sounds are more typical of problems in the lower airway.

Immobilize the neck and check for deformity, deviation, or an impaled object. Deviation may indicate a tension pneumothorax (see Chapter 4). Deformity would suggest a direct blow to the trachea with potential swelling and occlusion. Next, apply a cervical collar and continue manual stabilization.

Evaluation

Evaluation of the compromised airway should focus on the degree of blockage. In the conscious patient, complete obstruction may be evidenced by lack of air exchange, inability to speak or cough, and a hand on the throat (the universal sign of choking). In the unconscious patient, complete obstruction is indicated by resistance to artificial ventilation, inability to inflate the lungs, and gastric distention. Lack of breath sounds from the lungs is a sign that no air is being moved, but the reason is not always apparent.

Broken teeth (real or false), glass, metal, chewing gum, tobacco, food, and candy can all block the airway in trauma as well as nontrauma patients. Once you have identified the signs of airway distress, evaluate the degree and type of distress and respiratory compromise so that you can rapidly deliver appropriate care.

First, determine the location of the problem. Is it in the upper or lower airway? Are related injuries, such as a sucking chest wound, pneumothorax, or flail chest, contributing to respiratory distress? Are there extreme contributing factors, such as preexisting respiratory disease, entrapment, or position in the wreckage?

Aspiration is a major concern in lower airway compromise. The classic signs of respiratory distress will be present, but the telltale sounds will be lower (in the lung fields) than with upper airway problems, and can be diagnosed by listening to the chest with a stethoscope. Decreased chest movement and breath sounds may also be noted.

Caution!
Upper and lower airway problems may exhibit the same signs. Always check for the possibility of a combination of airway injuries.

Partial Obstruction. Patients with partial airway obstruction can be divided into two groups:

Partial obstruction with poor air exchange: These patients will be in severe respiratory distress, and will show several if not all of the symptoms previously noted. Air exchange is inadequate. Manage these patients immediately, as if they have *complete* airway obstruction, or they will deteriorate.

Partial obstruction with adequate air exchange: These patients may show anxiety and mild distress, but they can breathe adequately. They should have a good level of consciousness and color. Don't try to manually remove the obstruction. In transporting these patients, keep them as comfortable as possible and position them for easier breathing to the extent that their injuries will safely allow. These patients should have supplemental high-flow oxygen through a mask and be observed closely for any deterioration of their condition. If at any time their air exchange becomes inadequate, manage them as you would a victim with total airway obstruction.

It helps to know what is blocking the airway. You may have to suction liquids such as blood or vomitus, or you may need to turn the patient (while protecting the spine) onto her side. Solid obstruction may require you to apply abdominal thrusts or to remove the object with forceps, if you can do so safely and immediately and in accord with local protocols. An impaled object obstructing the airway presents one of the rare occasions where removal is indicated.

Complete Obstruction. Total blockage of the airway and lack of breathing may have any of several causes:

- obstruction by the tongue, broken teeth, saliva, or blood resulting from injuries to the upper airway
- direct trauma that crushes portions of the air passage or introduces a foreign body that may do so
- swelling of the airway as a result of trauma

A completely blocked airway is the highest treatment priority, since in four to six minutes irreparable brain damage will result.

Treatment

Visual examination, careful mechanical removal of foreign material, and suction may be all that are needed to open an obstructed airway. But some situations will challenge even the most experienced EMT.

No matter what method of airway management you use, be particularly careful to keep the neck and back immobilized, either by using devices for that purpose or by protecting the spine manually. Other methods of airway care, such as hyperextension or quickly turning the victim onto the side or stomach, always involve the possibility of spinal compromise. There are, however, many techniques and items of equipment that can help you accomplish such care.

Manual Methods of Airway Control. The tongue is the most common cause of partial or complete obstruction in an unconscious patient. Treatment consists of either of two maneuvers adapted from American Heart Association CPR guidelines:

1. The chin-lift method *without* head tilt: One rescuer pulls up on the patient's chin while a second person stabilizes the neck.
2. The jaw thrust: This maneuver can be performed by a single rescuer kneeling at the head of the patient. It involves pushing forward or upward at the angles of the jaw with the index and middle fingers while keeping the neck in traction with the hands and other fingers. *Note:* This second method is preferred since it allows you to open and evaluate the airway while securing the cervical spine.

Once you have opened the airway, package the patient by securing the cervical spine with a spineboard, straps, cervical collar, and a CID (cervical immobilization device) or padding and tape. Such immobilization will allow you to position the victim on his side if necessary to maintain a patent airway. Certainly immobilization is indicated for trauma patients in general because of this advantage of better airway control.

Managing the patient with complete airway obstruction. As desperate as this situation is, you still must attempt to protect the neck and spine of the patient. This will require you to alter standard techniques somewhat.

Open the airway using the techniques previously described, and attempt to ventilate. If complete obstruction is evident (from lack of chest expansion, resistance, and gastric distention), reposition the airway and attempt to ventilate once more. If still unsuccessful, stabilize the neck and inspect the airway. If you can see an obstruction and it is accessible, remove it. Be careful *not* to push the object deeper into the throat or to damage the throat.

If still unsuccessful, perform an abdominal thrust, inspect the mouth, and use a finger sweep to remove foreign matter if you can do so without pushing the obstruction deeper. Position the airway and attempt to ventilate. Repeat as many times as needed to open the airway.

Mechanical Means of Maintaining an Open Airway. Some important rules apply to the use of these aids.

- Equipment should be in good working order, ready for use, readily accessible, and appropriate for the patient.
- Be thoroughly familiar with the equipment, so that there is *no delay* or compromise in patient care.
- The availability of equipment is no excuse for delaying basic care of a patient. "Don't forget the basics!"

Oropharyngeal (oral) airway. This airway keeps the tongue from blocking the airway. Don't use it in a patient with a gag reflex, since it could cause vomiting and aspiration. Select the proper size of airway; the one most similar in length to the distance between the patient's earlobe and the corner of the mouth is best. If the airway is a big long, you can let the excess portion extend from the

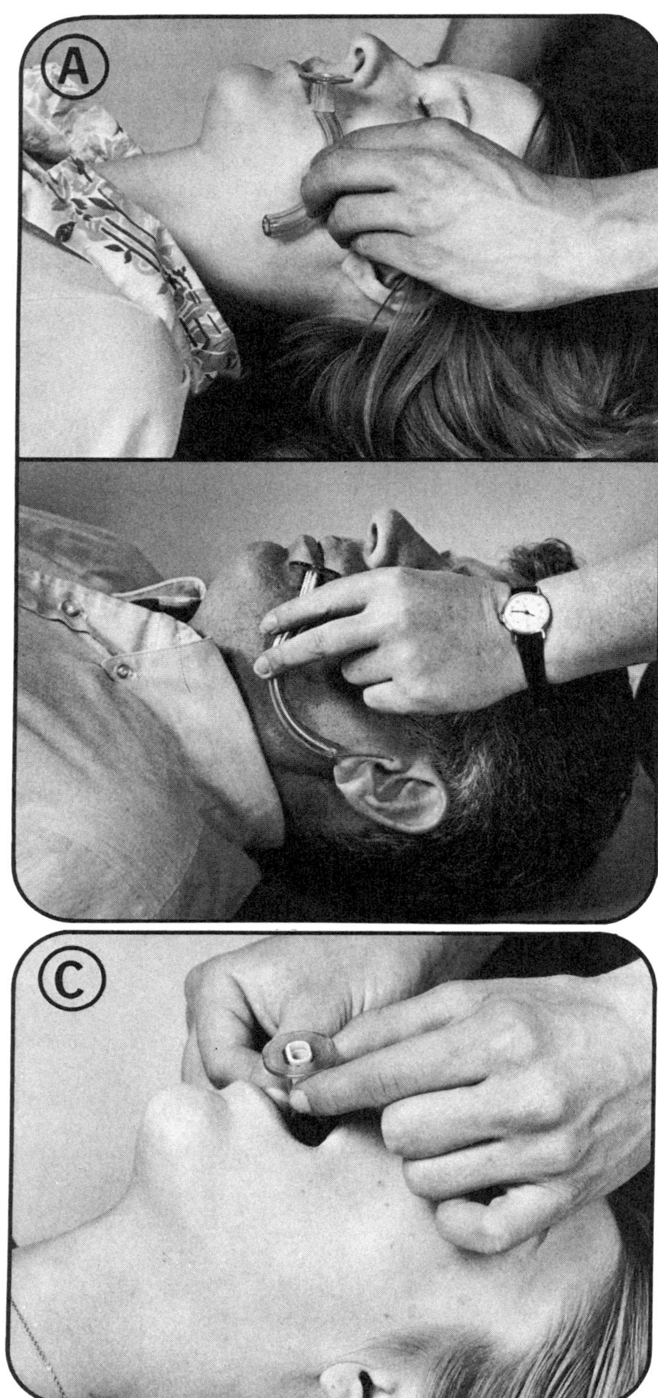

FIGURE 3.4 Use of oropharyngeal airway: (a) measure; (b) insert upside down; (c) rotate; (d) apply jaw thrust.

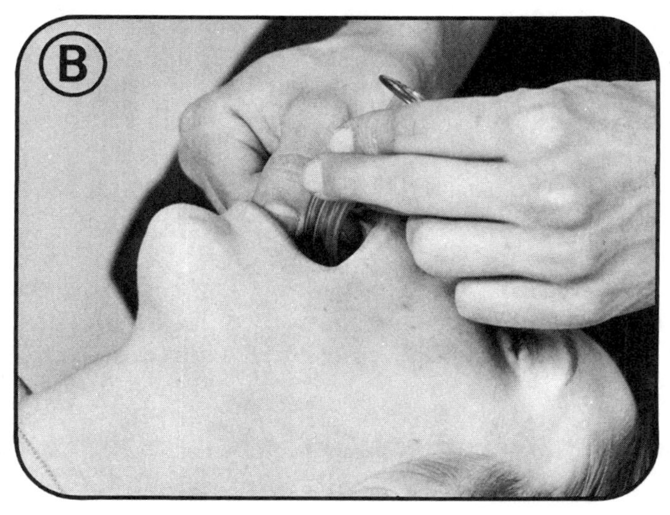
B

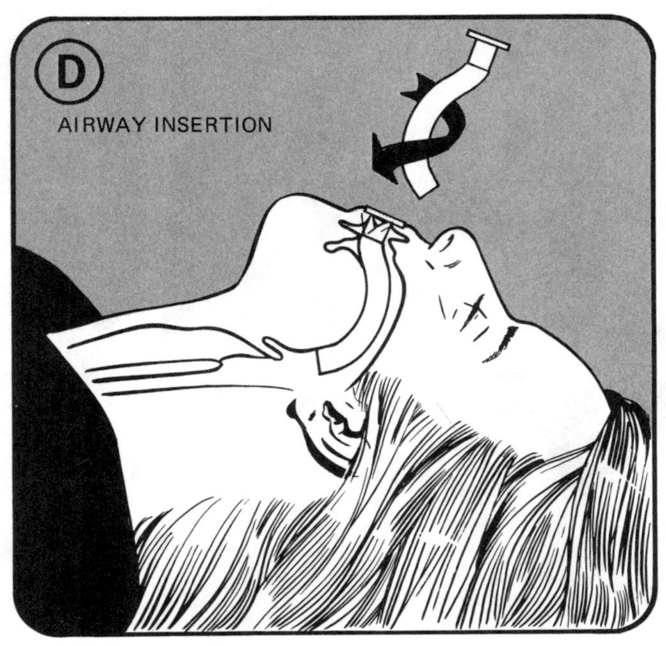
D
AIRWAY INSERTION

patient's mouth. Take extreme care when inserting the airway not to force the tongue or any other obstruction deeper into the throat. First inspect the mouth and make sure that no objects (including false teeth) are present. You can use one of two methods to insert the airway:

1. Hold the tongue in place with a tongue depressor as you insert the airway.
2. Open the mouth and introduce the airway upside down. Once the tip is beyond the tongue, rotate the airway 180 degrees into its normal position and slide it the rest of the way in. (Figure 3.4)

Nasopharyngeal airway. In some cases, especially in patients with some remaining gag reflex, or where the patient's mouth is clenched shut, this airway may be especially useful (Figure 3.5). Select the size the same as you would for the oral airway. Apply a surgical lubricant to the tube before inserting it. Turn the airway so that the bevel is toward the nasal septum and gently in-

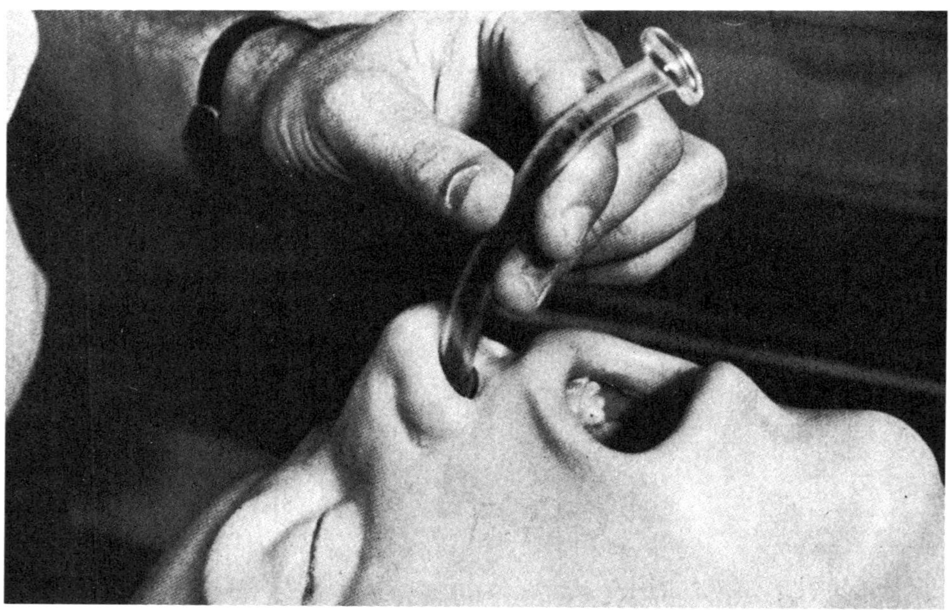

FIGURE 3.5 Use of nasopharyngeal airway: (a) measure; (b) lubricate; (c) insert straight back.

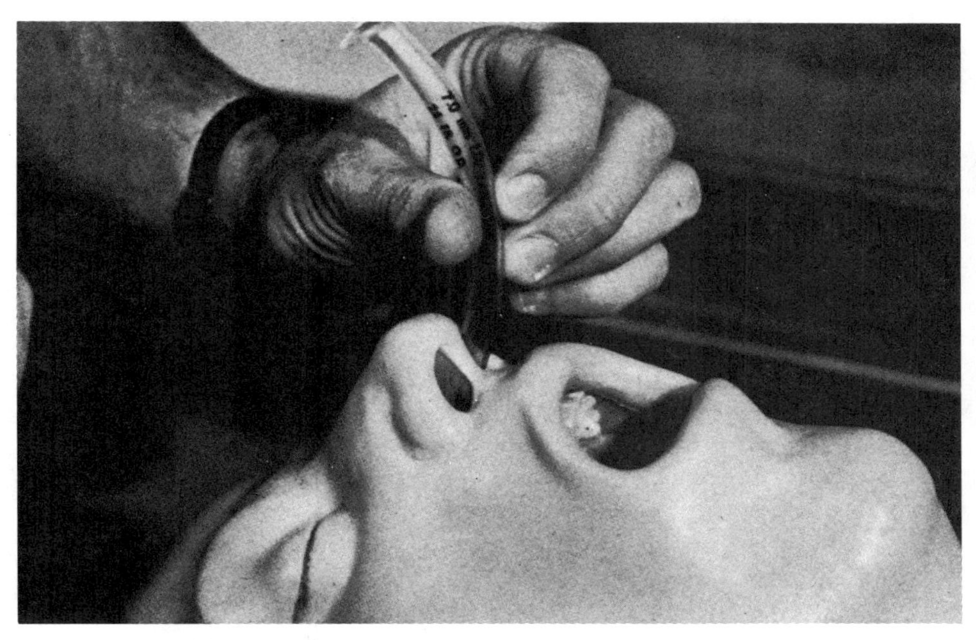

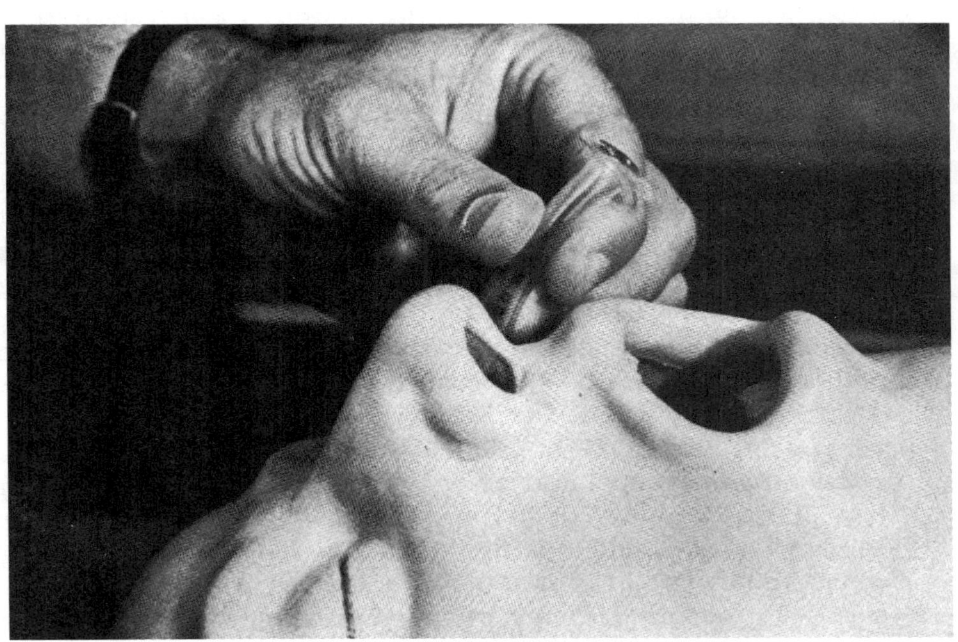

sert the tube straight back (as if paralleling the roof of the mouth). If you encounter resistance, withdraw the airway slightly and introduce it again. If there is still resistance, try inserting the tube into the other nares. *Never* force the nasal airway. As with the oral airway, if coughing and gagging occur, withdraw the tube. Use special care if facial fractures exist.

Suction devices. Suctioning is a vital aid in keeping the airway clear. Not only can foreign matter compromise the airway and produce hypoxia, but aspiration often produces long-term complications such as pneumonia that can be life-threatening.

Field suction devices have greatly improved in recent years and now provide adequate suction capacity and battery duration. Suction tip devices have also been improved. You should have a thorough working knowledge of the device. As with all equipment, you should check the unit and have it ready for use during each shift.

Prepare the suction device before introducing it into the patient, to avoid extended periods of hypoventilation. In selecting the type of tip, consider the viscosity of the material to be suctioned. If you select a catheter, the size should be based on the patient's size and the route to be used (oral or nasal). If solids need to be removed, the wide-bore tonsil tip is preferred. It is suggested that all suction tips have a thumb control since this allows the tip to be introduced while the suction is off, without robbing the patient of oxygen.

Suctioning should take 10 seconds or less so that the patient does not become hypoxic. The general rule is to suction for as short a time as needed to clear the airway. If possible, hyperventilate the patient *before* and *after* suctioning. Also, avoid introducing the tip so deeply that it touches the larynx. Introduce the catheter no deeper than the distance between the patient's earlobe and the corner of the mouth (as in measuring for an oral airway).

The most obvious complication to be avoided in suctioning is hypoxia. Prolonged suctioning will rob the patient of oxygen. Suctioning too deeply may stimulate the vagus nerves, which in turn slows the pulse—something your patient may ill afford.

If possible, avoid making the patient gag during suctioning since this may produce vomiting and/or increase intracranial pressure (ICP). Increased ICP is especially undesirable in a patient with a head injury. Exercise extreme caution in nasal suctioning patients with head and facial trauma. Certain fractures may allow the catheter to end up inside the skull.

Caution!
Medical Control in some areas may not allow the use of nasal airways or nasal suctioning. Know your local protocol before practicing these techniques.

VENTILATION

After you have cleared obstructions and the airway is open, you must ensure adequate ventilation. If the patient is ventilating adequately, monitor him or her closely (keeping the airway open).

Seriously injured patients with respiratory distress or potential for shock should receive supplemental oxygen. In general, you should provide a flow of 10 to 15 liters per minute using the best means available to deliver the highest concentration possible. Several alternatives are available; the choice depends on the patient's condition and injuries.

1. The *nasal cannula* delivers oxygen at a concentration of around 35 percent. It allows the patient to communicate easily with emergency personnnel and does not create a smothering sensation in some apprehensive patients. Don't use it if you want a higher oxygen concentration or if the patient's condition prevents breathing through the nose.
2. The *nonrebreathing mask* delivers 90 to 100 percent concentration and is excellent for patients needing higher oxygen levels. The disadvantage of this and any mask is that some patients will not tolerate the restrictive feeling it gives them. Masks also interfere with oral communication between you and the patient.
3. The *partial-rebreathing mask* mixes more ambient air with the oxygen, thereby reducing oxygen concentration to 70 to 90 percent.
4. The Veni (Venturi) mask, while more complicated, allows delivery of a precise oxygen concentration, which may be desirable in some medical emergencies but is rarely necessary in the trauma setting.

If the patient is not breathing, or if respirations are inadequate, you must provide ventilation. Remember, just because respiratory efforts are visible does not mean ventilation is adequate—look at the patient's overall condition to decide. Assisted ventilations coordinated with and/or added to the patient's own ventilations may be needed. Other patients may require complete ventilatory resuscitation. In either case, you can use one of the following techniques.

1. Mouth-to-Mouth or Mouth-to-Nose Ventilation. This is the simplest and quickest way to ventilate a patient. It requires no equipment and is sufficient to maintain the patient. An obvious disadvantage is possible exposure to communicable disease.

2. Mouth-to-Mask Ventilation. Because of AIDS and other communicable diseases, the resuscitation mask offers some reassurance to the rescuer. Masks not only provide an easy and effective alternative to mouth-to-mouth, but allow the use of supplemental oxygen. The use of an oral airway with the resuscitation mask further improves its effectiveness (Figure 3.6).

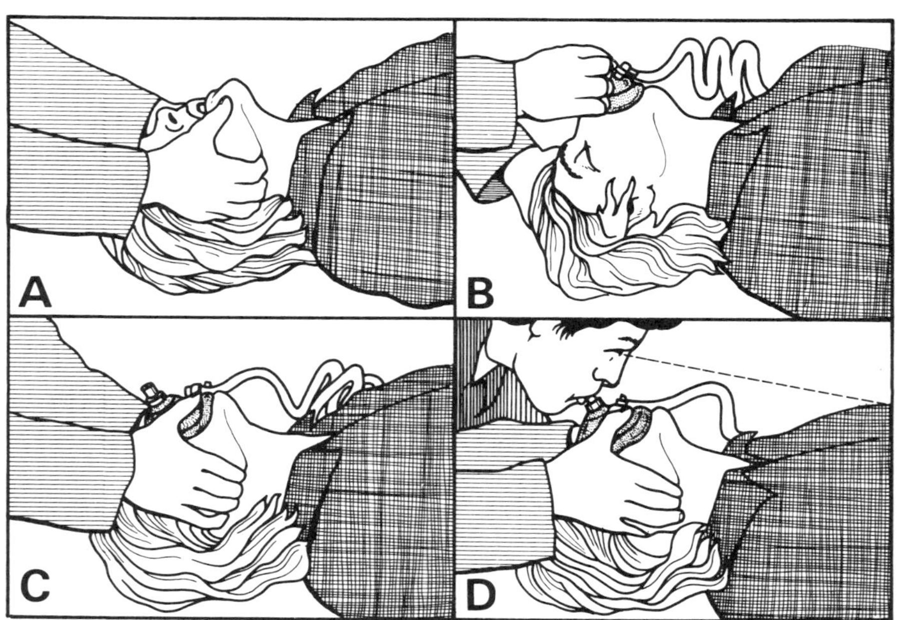

FIGURE 3.6 Proper mouth-to-mask ventilation.

3. Bag-Valve-Mask (BVM) Resuscitation. BMVs are extremely difficult to use effectively because it is almost impossible to maintain an adequate seal between the mask and the patient's face with one hand. Many believe the technique requires *two* rescuers. For this reason, it is recommended that a BVM *not* be used as a single-rescuer technique unless an endotracheal tube is in place. And even then, you must be well enough trained so that you do not compromise the patient's spine. Choose the BVM only if you can achieve adequate ventilation and only if you are extremely proficient in its use. Finally, the use of a BVM requires the introduction of an oral or nasal airway and supplemental oxygen.

4. Resuscitation with a Positive-Pressure Ventilator. This device is useful with breathing patients because its demand valve allows delivery of very high concentrations of oxygen when the patient inhales. Positive pressure can be used in the nonbreathing patient, but there still is the problem of maintaining an adequate seal between the mask to the patient's face. Moreover, positive-pressure ventilation in the presence of pneumothorax can be dangerous.

In addition, there are several new airway devices on the market that are reported to provide an open airway and carry minimal risk in application. These devices may prove to be valuable in prehospital care, but they require specialized training as well as state and local approval.

CONCLUSION

Airway management is job number one for the EMT. Providing adequate oxygenation is the top priority in all forms of trauma, because inadequate ventilation or airway compromise can kill quickly. Know how to assess the airway and ventilation and how to manage conditions that threaten both.

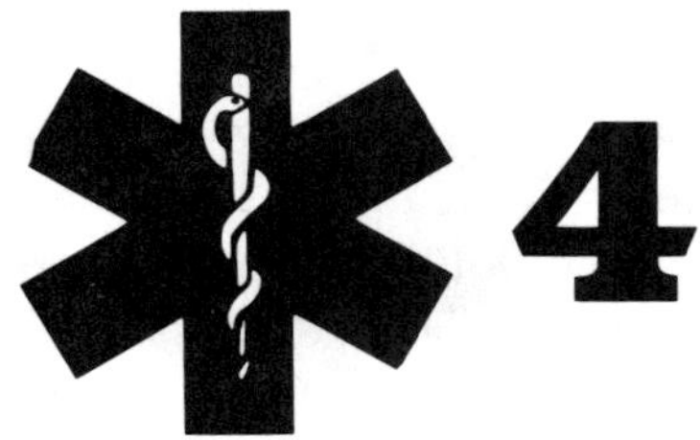

Thoracic Trauma

INTRODUCTION

Injuries to the chest account for about 25 percent of all trauma deaths and represent an important challenge for the EMT, since emergency medical intervention may be lifesaving. As with all trauma patients, (1) airway, (2) breathing, and (3) circulation must be evaluated in every patient with blunt or penetrating chest trauma. Virtually all types of chest trauma have hypoxia (systemic lack of oxygen) as a common feature. The hypoxia is often compounded by hypovolemic shock from hemorrhage and will be life-threatening if not rapidly corrected. Hypoxia is usually the result of abnormal airway pressure relationships—tension pneumothorax and sucking chest wounds are good examples—or is caused by direct injury to the lung itself, as in pulmonary contusion.

The treatment principles of oxygen administration and correction of shock apply to all patients with chest injuries. However, there are also specific treatments, discussed later in the chapter, for each type of chest injury.

As is true for trauma to other body parts, injuries to the thorax may be classified as either penetrating or blunt. Penetrating injuries are usually due to gunshot or stab wounds but may be caused by the more dramatic impalement injuries. Penetrating injuries to the chest are usually manifested in a pneumothorax, hemothorax, or sucking chest wound.

Blunt injury to the chest is more common and usually follows motor vehicle crashes. Signs and symptoms of blunt injuries to the chest may be more subtle than those of penetrating trauma, but these injuries are equally life-threatening and usually demand greater skill in early diagnosis.

OBJECTIVES

At the completion of this chapter, you will be able to:

1. Recognize the major features of chest anatomy and physiology.
2. Define terms used to describe major chest injuries.
3. Explain the significance of the symptoms and signs of chest trauma.
4. Identify serious chest injuries and explain the appropriate emergency medical management.

ANATOMY OF THE THORAX

The thorax (chest) is the upper portion of the human torso. It is bounded by the neck above and the abdomen below, and is a semi-rigid structure formed by the rib cage, the sternum in front, and the thoracic spine in back. The upper portion is further protected by the heavy muscles of the shoulder girdle and the clavicles. The thorax may be internally divided into the pleural spaces (the membrane-lined sacs, one on each side, containing the lungs) and the mediastinum. The mediastinum, in the middle of the chest, contains the heart and the great blood vessels emerging from and returning to it—the aorta and vena cava and the pulmonary arteries and pulmonary veins. The mediastinum also contains the trachea and the esophagus. The thorax is separated from the abdomen by the thin muscular structure of the diaphragm, which on exhalation may arch as high as the fifth rib anteriorly. The liver and the spleen are within the thoracic portion of the abdomen and are frequently injured in blunt thoracic trauma.

COMMON TERMS

1. *cyanosis:* the bluish discoloration about the lips, face, and nail beds associated with lack of oxygen and caused by desaturation of hemoglobin (usually a late sign of chest injury)
2. *dyspnea:* difficult or painful breathing; common to most severe chest injuries

3. *hemoptysis:* the coughing up of blood
4. *paradoxical chest movement:* the inward movement on inspiration and outward movement on expiration of a segment of the chest wall under which ribs have been fractured in more than one place
5. *pleuritic pain:* pain resulting from irritation of the membranes lining the lung; worsened by taking a deep breath or coughing
6. *subcutaneous emphysema:* air in the soft tissue of the chest wall that, on palpation, feels like Rice Crispies under the skin; may indicate injury to the lung, trachea, or bonchus.
7. *tachypnea:* rapid respiratory rate (greater than 20 breaths per minute)

LIFE-THREATENING CHEST INJURIES

Tension Pneumothorax

Tension pneumothorax results from increased pressure in the pleural space around one lung. The pressure collapses that lung and pushes the mediastinum toward the other lung, partially obstructing ventilation (Figure 4.1). Tension pneumothorax, by pushing on the vena cava, also interferes with the return of venous blood to the heart. All these effects have the disastrous result of hypoxia combined with low cardiac output. Tension pneumothorax is usually produced by damage to the lung tissue or the major airways such that air is released into the pleural space but has no means of escape. Therefore, pressure builds inside the space. The condition has been likened to a one-way valve producing abnormal pressure in the chest.

The signs and symptoms of tension pneumothorax will depend in part on the mechanism of the wound. Every patient with tension pneumothorax, however, will be dyspneic and will usually exhibit severe respiratory distress. The patient commonly will be tachypneic, and tachycardia will result with the usual signs and symptoms of shock. As with all physical examinations, *look, listen,* and *feel.* The breath sounds on the affected side will usually be markedly diminished or absent. In severe cases, the trachea, palpable in the suprasternal notch low in the anterior neck, will be displaced away from the side of the tension. The neck veins will be distended if the patient is not in severe hypovolemic shock.

As with all severe injuries, begin initial management of a patient with tension pneumothorax by ensuring an open airway, ad-

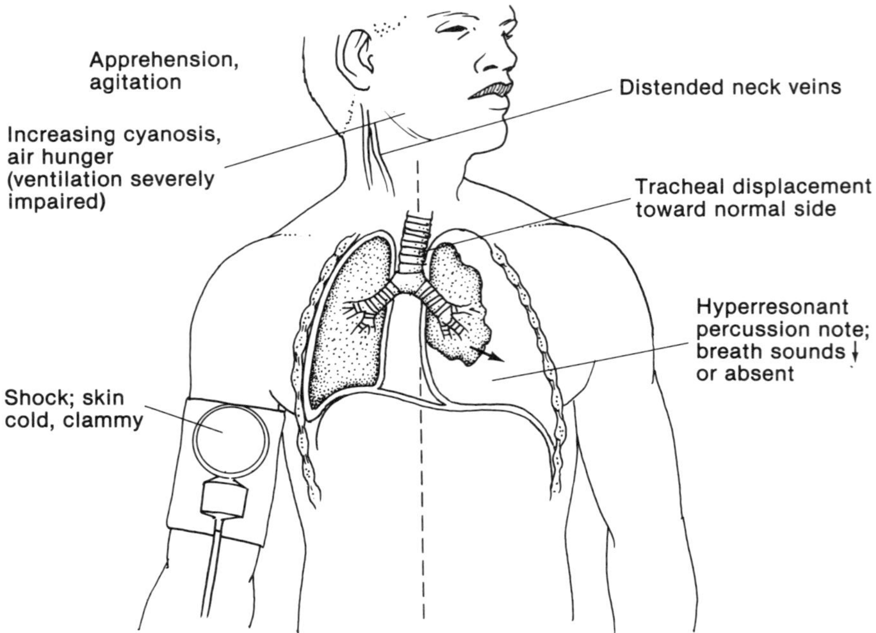

FIGURE 4.1 Tension pneumothorax.

ministering a high flow of oxygen, and the correcting hypovolemic shock by controlling any external hemorrhage.

> **Caution!**
> Inflating the abdominal portion of the PASG may aggravate the respiratory distress of the patient with pneumothorax.

Open Pneumothorax (Sucking Chest Wound)

Sucking chest wounds are most commonly produced by large-bore weapons, shotgun blasts, or impalement injuries. If the diameter of the opening into the chest is greater than two-thirds that of the trachea, air may enter the chest through the sucking wound rather than through the tracheobronchial tree (Figure 4.2). The life-threatening effects of this injury are obvious.

The assessment of open pneumothorax is usually obvious, and the injury to the chest wall may be combined with severe internal injuries to the lungs or to the large blood vessels of the medi-

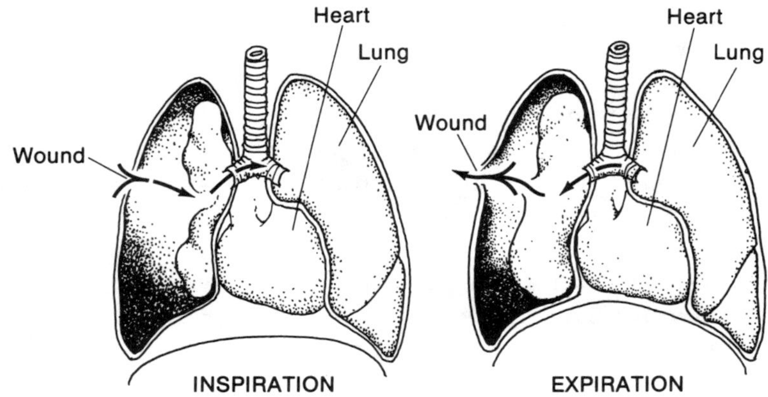

FIGURE 4.2 Open pneumothorax.

astinum. Unless you inspect or palpate the patient's entire chest, you may miss an open pneumothorax in the lateral or posterior areas of the chest.

The emergency management of an open pneumothorax involves covering the defect so the patient will be able to ventilate normally through the airway. This is best accomplished with a sterile covering such as the aluminum-foil inside of a Vaseline gauze packet. This covering has enough Vaseline on it to be sticky and is about the right size for most injuries. Take care when securing this covering over the wound to tape it on only three sides. That way, should tension pneumothorax develop within the chest, there will be a flutter-valve mechanism on the untaped side to allow air to escape and not be drawn back into the chest when the patient inspires.

Caution!
Tension pneumothorax may occur following emergency management of open pneumothorax, regardless of the mechanism used to secure the dressing. If so, momentarily remove the dressing to release pressure.

Flail Chest

Flail chest is an unstable segment of the chest wall produced by the fracture of several ribs in at least two places. As a result of the fractures, the flail segment has no bony union with the rest of the chest wall. Flail chest follows blunt trauma and usually indicates severe injury. The lung underlying the flail segment is commonly bruised, and the resulting pulmonary contusion is responsible for the most severe effects of flail chest. During inspiration and expiration, the flail segment moves parodoxically—that is, on inspiration it moves inward and on expiration it moves outward (Figure 4.3).

The patient who is conscious will experience pain and tenderness in the area of the rib fractures. There may be palpable subcutaneous emphysema if the lung has been penetrated, and paradoxical chest wall mount will be apparent in many instances. Dyspnea and tachypnea are usually present. A pneumothorax or hemothorax may be present as well as many other injuries.

The usual supportive measures of airway maintenance and shock correction are extremely important. Some authorities have advocated stabilizing flail segment with sandbags and tape or transporting the patient with the flail segment down. However, these maneuvers take time, are not very effective, and may endanger patients with potential spinal injury. They also make airway management more difficult. The patient should be transported in a supine position for better monitoring and emergency treatment en route. Oxygen therapy is always indicated.

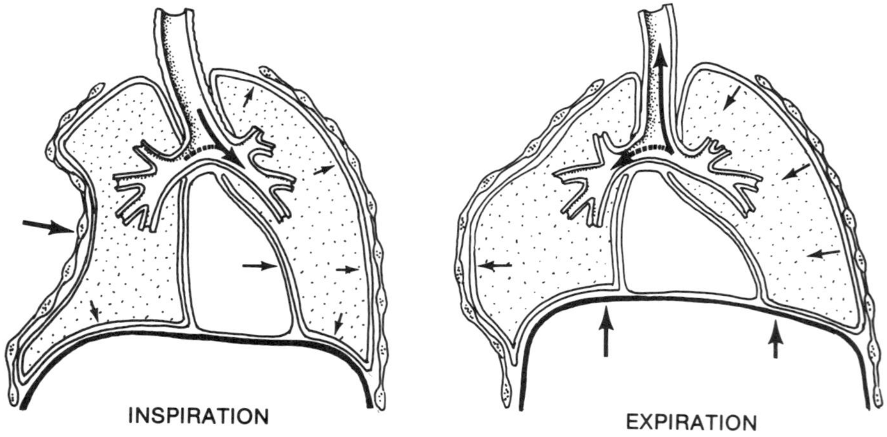

FIGURE 4.3 Paradoxical motion of the chest wall. Compare with normal respiration, illustrated in FIGURE 3.3.

Impalement Injuries

These injuries are produced by a variety of penetrating objects, most commonly the knife. Motor vehicle crashes may cause impalement by a variety of objects, ranging from rear-view mirrors to steering wheels, fence posts, and even guardrails. Impalement may produce a variety of chest injuries, such as massive hemothorax, flail segments, open sucking chest wounds, or even cardiac tamponade. Despite the dramatic appearance of these patients, many of them are salvageable with proper early management. The hallmark of therapy for an impalement injury is to transport the patient with the impaled object stabilized and in place if this is at all possible. Extrication will often require complex equipment, including metal or wood saws. The temptation to remove the impaled object for ease of extrication should be resisted, since the object may be preventing major bleeding. Removal could therefore result in fatal hemorrhage. A sucking chest wound next to an impaled object should be treated as previously described.

Diaphragmatic Rupture

The diaphragm may be ruptured by either blunt or penetrating trauma. Most diaphragmatic ruptures that cause early symptoms are the result of blunt trauma. Blunt trauma to the abdomen may cause a sudden increase in intra-abdominal pressure and a sudden upward thrusting of the diaphragm. A rupture may occur on either side but is more common on the left, because the liver appears to offer some protection to the right side. Herniation of abdominal contents into the chest causes impairment of ventilation, mediastinal shift, and significant hypoxia (Figure 4.4).

Signs and Symptoms. The signs and symptoms of diaphragmatic rupture may be very difficult to detect, even for an experienced physician. As more and more of the abdominal contents are forced up into the chest cavity, the breath sounds on the affected side diminish and a pneumothorax or hemothorax may be suspected. As with all serious chest injuries, the patient will experience moderate to severe respiratory distress with tachypnea and dyspnea. Abdominal tenderness or chest wall tenderness is common.

There is no prehospital emergency medical care for a ruptured

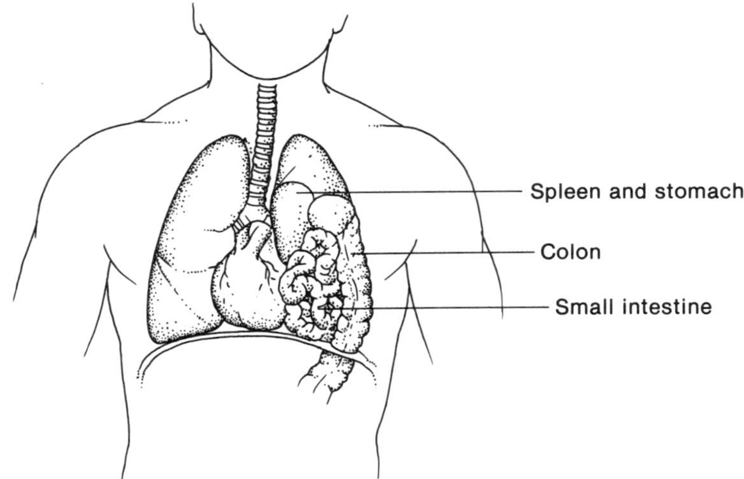

FIGURE 4.4 Rupture of left hemidiaphragm with herniation of abdominal contents.

diaphragm. Follow the general principles of airway maintenance, adequate oxygenation and ventilation, and the correction of hypovolemic shock.

Caution!
Inflation of the abdominal compartment of the PASG causes further herniation of abdominal contents into the chest and marked alterations in intrathoracic pressure. With most chest injuries, avoid inflation of the abdominal portion of the PASG.

Massive Hemothorax

Massive hemothorax may result from either blunt or penetrating trauma to the chest and is commonly due to laceration of the large blood vessels to the lung or the blood vessels of the chest wall. In a massive hemothorax, more than 1500 cc of blood is present in one pleural space. The patient is suffering from hypovolemic shock and respiratory distress since the lung on the affected side will be partially or completely collapsed by the blood (Figure 4.5).

Virtually all patients with massive hemothorax will have signs and symptoms of hypovolemic shock. Tachypnea, tachycardia, and

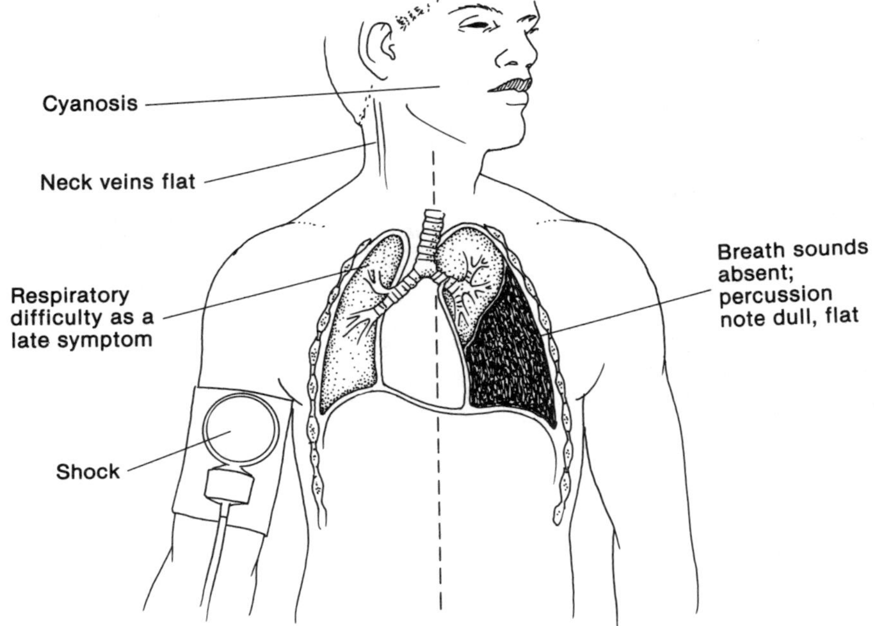

FIGURE 4.5 Massive hemothorax.

dyspnea are almost always present. Breath sounds may be diminished to absent, and the percussion note is dull. The trachea is usually not deviated in the suprasternal notch, and the neck veins are usually flat rather than distended.

Bleeding into the chest cannot be controlled or treated in the field. Provide an adequate airway, oxygenate, and immediately transport.

Massive hemothorax and tension pneumothorax may be easily confused, and a needle decompression of a massive hemothorax should cause no ill effects to the patient. General supportive measures for tension pneumothorax and hemothorax are the same.

Cardiac Tamponade

Cardiac tamponade is the result of blood rapidly accumulating in the pericardial sac (Figure 4.6). As little as 75 to 100 cc may produce significant symptoms. Cardiac tamponade is usually the result of penetrating trauma of the chest. However, it may be produced in some cases by blunt trauma tearing a portion of the heart

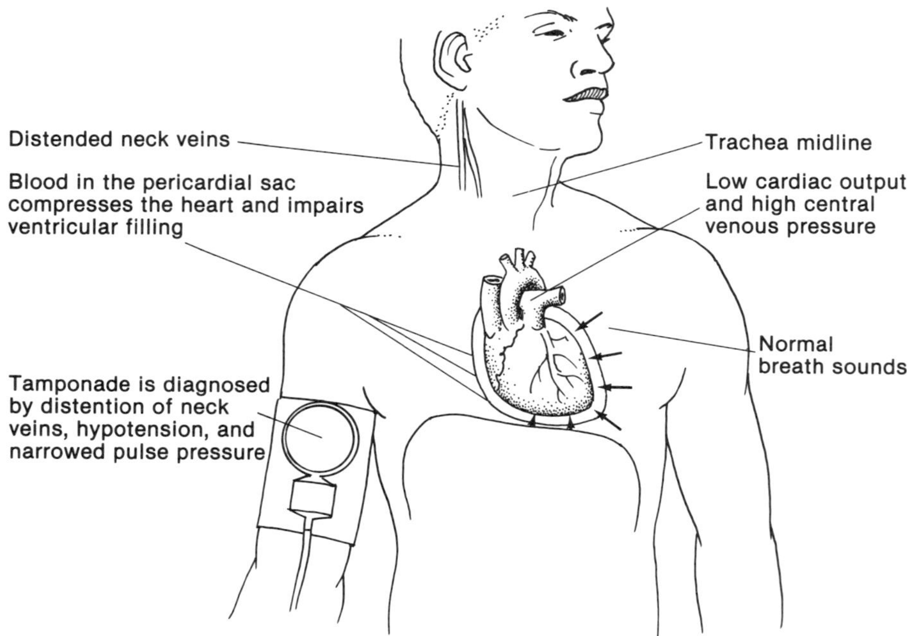

FIGURE 4.6 Cardiac tamponade.

or the great vessels inside the pericardium. The blood in the pericardial sac will not allow the heart to relax and fill with blood, remarkably diminishing cardiac output.

In a patient who is alert, anxiety combined with tachypnea and tachycardia may create a feeling of "impending doom." The heart tones are classically muffled (an unreliable sign in the field), breath sounds are normal, and the neck veins may be distended. The usual signs of shock will also be present. Pulse pressure diminishes as systolic and diastolic pressure differences decrease.

Manage patients with cardiac tamponade by establishing an airway and providing adequate oxygenation. Despite distended neck veins and the appearance of adequate blood volume, intravenous access and cystalloid infusion are indicated.

Cardiac Contusion

A cardiac contusion is a bruise of the heart muscle resulting from blunt trauma. It results from deceleration injuries, especially if the chest is injured by the steering wheel. The effects of cardiac contusion may not be initially apparent unless there has been severe damage to the heart muscle or rupture of internal heart structures.

The signs and symptoms of cardiac contusion may be difficult or impossible to determine in the field. The patient will usually have pain over the anterior chest. He may have a fractured sternum, fractured ribs, or an obvious contusion of the chest wall. There may be initial rhythm disturbances apparent on the cardiac monitor. There is no specific emergency medical care for cardiac contusion other than adequate oxygenation and ventilation and prevention of hypovolemic shock.

Traumatic Asphyxia

Traumatic asphyxia is caused by a massive crushing injury to the chest and upper torso. It is commonly the result of a cave-in injury, but it may also be produced by motor vehicle crashes or industrial accidents. The increase in intrathoracic pressure may cause other injuries, including pneumothorax, flail chest, cardiac contusion, or cardiac tamponade. The application of pressure will prevent the patient from breathing adequately, for the chest cavity cannot expand during inspiration.

The patient will show signs of increased vascular pressure in the head and neck. There may be hemorrhages or bulging in the conjunctiva of the eyes (Figure 4.7). There may be a reddish or bluish discoloration of the face and neck, and the neck veins may be distended. The patient will be anxious and may have severe respiratory distress or signs of hypovolemic shock. In other instances, despite a rather frightful appearance, the patient may be in little or no distress.

Establish an adequate airway immediately and administer high-flow oxygen. Treat associated chest injuries as previously described. Promptly transport the victim to a facility prepared to care for severe trauma.

Potentially Life-Threatening Chest Injuries

You will encounter many chest injuries that are less severe than those just mentioned. However, they may be life-threatening if not recognized. A simple pneumothorax that is not under tension may produce significant symptoms of respiratory difficulty, especially in patients with preexisting lung disease. Patients with a simple

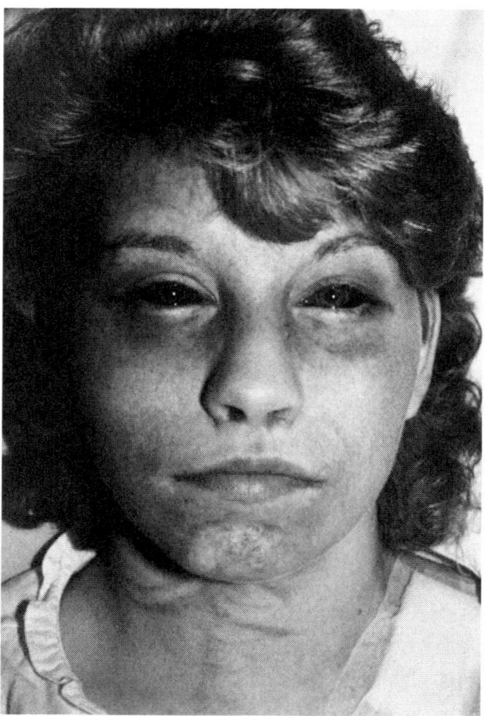

FIGURE 4.7 Traumatic asphyxia.

pneumothorax will frequently be dyspneic and have chest pain on the affected side; breath sounds will be diminished to absent. The neck veins will not be distended and the trachea will not be deviated, as they are in a tension pneumothorax.

Subcutaneous emphysema may be very dramatic and may extend from the patient's head to the lower extremities. The condition by itself seldom produces severe symptoms. However, subcutaneous emphysema may indicate pneumothorax or tension pneumothorax and suggests trauma to the lungs or airways.

Rib fractures commonly follow blunt trauma to the chest. The patient will always experience pain at the fracture site and will usually self-splint her chest. Avoid taping the ribs or using cravats. Transport the patient to the hospital, where other, potentially more serious injuries may be sought.

There are other intrathoracic injuries that may not be recognized in the field, such as blunt rupture of the esophagus and incomplete tears of the thoracic aorta. It is very important to supply the treating physician with the circumstances of the accident, since many of these injuries will be suspected based on the mechanism of injury.

CONCLUSION

Chest trauma causes one in every four trauma deaths. If the airway is patent and the patient continues to have breathing difficulty or chest pain, chest trauma is likely. Provide oxygen and transport the patient quickly to a medical facility prepared to treat patients with chest trauma.

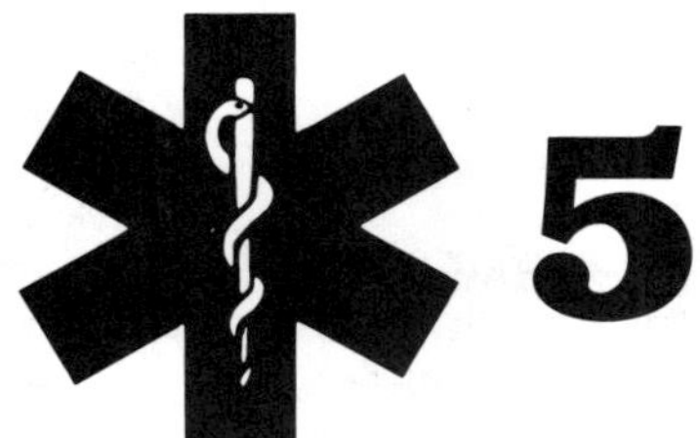

5 Shock

INTRODUCTION

Shock is a state of inadequate tissue perfusion that, untreated, leads to irreversible changes and death. Shock has been termed a momentary pause in the act of dying. Prompt recognition and management of shock is a major responsibility of the EMT. Recognition of shock is essential in determining the urgency of care, the proper facility for definitive care, and the mode of transport.

OBJECTIVES

At the completion of this chapter, you should be able to:

1. Define shock.
2. Describe the major types of shock and their pathophysiologic differences.
3. Describe the findings common to all forms of shock and explain proper field intervention.
4. State the dynamic relationship among the heart, blood vessels, and blood volume in maintaining perfusion to the tissues.
5. Describe how the pneumatic antishock garment (PASG) elevates blood pressure and explain the indications and contraindications to its use.

PATHOPHYSIOLOGY

Normal perfusion requires an intact cardiovascular system and adequate oxygen exchange. In most types of shock, poor perfusion is due to a failure of the cardiovascular system. This system can be thought of as having three parts: the heart (pump), the blood vessels (pipes), and the blood.

Epinephrine and norepinephrine control the heart, by increasing the rate and force of its contractions. These effects are balanced by the vagus nerves, which tend to slow the heart rate. The strength of contraction and the heart rate can be varied in order to increase or decrease cardiac output. These modifications in heart rate and contractility are accomplished early and automatically.

If cardiac contraction is strong and blood volume is normal, the pulse is slow. If cardiac contraction is weakened and blood volume is normal, an increase in cardiac rate can compensate to ensure an adequate cardiac output.

However, if blood volume is reduced (by bleeding, for example), both the heart and the blood vessels must respond. The heart rate and force of contractility increase and the force of peripheral circulation increases (vasoconstriction). Cardiac output can also be influenced by medications and by external circumstances such as fright, heat, or cold.

The blood vessels are the tubes that carry the blood to and from the tissues of the body. These include arteries, arterioles, capillaries, venules, and veins (Figure 5.1). The arteries and arterioles have muscular walls that are controlled by the autonomic nervous system. The capacity of the capillary beds in various tissues can be controlled by relaxing or constricting these muscles. The body can open certain tissues to flow while closing others, depending upon the specific circumstances and needs at a given time. Stimuli that cause these changes include need of an organ for oxygen, need to clear metabolic wastes, fright, and temperature.

Normal adult blood volume is about six liters. Fluid can move to some extent into and out of the vascular system in order to maintain an adequate intravascular blood volume. The heart normally pumps about six liters a minute to maintain blood supply throughout the body.

Certain organs require a continuous high rate of perfusion; other tissues have intermittent demands for high flow rates. The

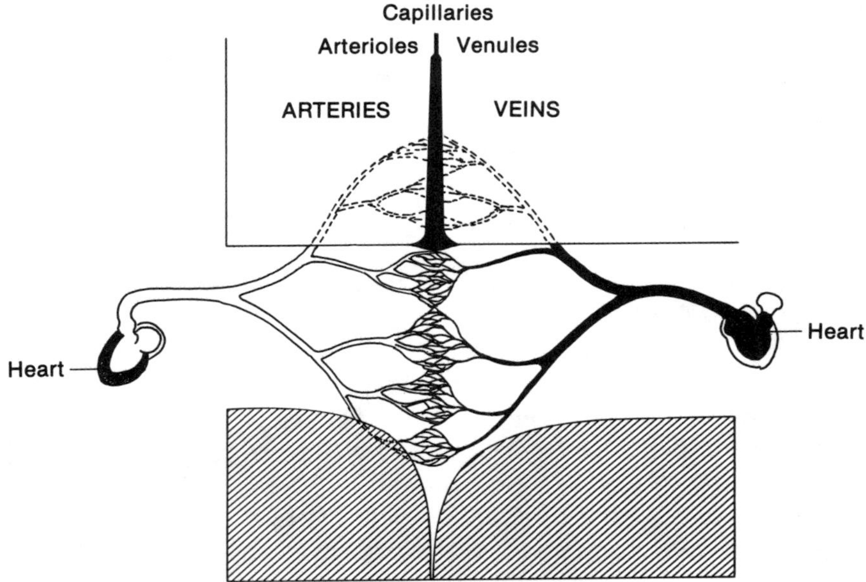

FIGURE 5.1 The circulatory system.

vascular system is constantly adjusting in order to meet these needs. In shock states the blood is shunted to the brain, heart, and lungs at the expense of other tissues. The heart requires continuous perfusion in order to pump. The brain and spinal cord begin to sustain permanent damage to nerve cells after 4 to 6 minutes of impaired flow. The kidney will develop permanent damage after about 45 minutes of inadequate perfusion. Skeletal muscles can tolerate ischemia for only one or two hours. No tissue in the body is immune to damage from poor perfusion. Reestablishment of tissue perfusion with oxygenated blood is therefore essential to the treatment of shock.

There are several types of shock, but only four causes (which may be present in various combinations in the trauma patient):

1. Inadequate pump (heart failure)
2. Overdilation of the vascular system (loss of vascular tone)
3. Inadequate blood volume (hypovolemia)
4. Inadequate oxygenation of the blood (respiratory failure)

Regardless of the cause, the effect of shock is the same. Poor tissue perfusion results in insufficient oxygen and nutrients, and metabolic waste products accumulate. If this state is not corrected, the patient dies.

SIGNS AND SYMPTOMS

Shock is progressive; it develops in stages. Early recognition is vital, but the signs and symptoms can be subtle in the early stages. Assume that the patient at risk has or will develop shock, and manage accordingly. The degree of shock will vary with time, the severity of insult, and preexisting conditions. Be particularly alert when dealing with the elderly, young children, pregnant women, and patients with preexisting illness.

Many factors can influence the severity of shock. Hypothermia or hyperthermia can predispose the patient to shock. Starved, poorly nourished, or water-deprived patients are most susceptible to shock. Excessive fatigue or pain can increase the severity of shock. Shock can be aggravated by delays in management and by inappropriate or rough handling.

Symptoms of shock include weakness, dizziness, thirst, coolness, nausea, and fearfulness. Do not expect to see all of these in a given patient or at one time. Patients in shock may have an obvious source of external blood loss or more subtle signs of internal bleeding. They may be restless and vomiting. Their level of consciousness may deteriorate. The pulse may be rapid and weak and the blood pressure may fall. Respirations can be rapid, weak, labored or possibly gasping. The patient may be pallid and sweating. Their eyes may be dull, with dilated pupils. They may exhibit cyanosis of the lips and mucous membranes. Poor capillary refill is possible.

In the early stages of shock, expect to see anxiety and an increase in pulse and respirations. These are compensatory mechanisms for enhancing tissue perfusion. As the patient begins to worsen, the following signs and symptoms may be present: pallor, sweating, cyanosis, a rapid and weak pulse, labored respirations, weakness, thirst, and nausea. Severe, late shock is marked by loss of consciousness, hypotension, a weak and thready pulse, and weak or gasping respirations. A fall in blood pressure is also a late sign of shock.

Caution!
Hypotension signals that the body's compensatory mechanisms have been exhausted. Do not wait for a falling blood pressure to manage a patient in shock.

GENERAL MANAGEMENT

There are some general measures that apply to all types of shock:

1. Establish an airway. Remember to protect the C-spine while doing so. A patient who is talking or shouting has an adequate airway.
2. Give oxygen. Shock results in poor oxygenation at the tissue level, and patients in shock have an increased oxygen requirement. Give high-concentration oxygen by the most appropriate means.
3. *Stop hemorrhage!* If the patient is bleeding externally, apply pressure to control it. Internal bleeding requires definitive operative care in most instances.
4. Do not administer anything by mouth. Patients in shock are prone to aspiration and may require surgery. Do not give anything to eat or drink even if a patient complains of thirst.
5. Maintain normal temperature. Prevent heat loss with blankets over and under the patient, but don't heat the patient.
6. Minimize pain. Avoid unnecessary and rough handling. Splint fractures to decrease further blood loss and pain. Immobilize the patient with care.
7. Monitor the patient. Blood pressure, pulse, respirations and level of consciousness need to be monitored continuously and recorded every five minutes.
8. Transport immediately. Definitive treatment is the key to survival with patients in shock. Transport quickly and efficiently to the site of definitive care.

THE PNEUMATIC ANTISHOCK GARMENT (PASG)

The PASG—also known as military antishock trousers (MAST), external counterpressure, or the G suit) is a three-chambered device that is applied about the legs and abdomen of the victim (Figure 5.2). Through a series of valves, the PASG can be inflated in the adult to a pressure above mean arterial pressure. Although early users attributed the beneficial effects of PASG use to central shunting of blood from the lower half of the body, subsequent research has demonstrated the rise in blood pressure to be due to an increase in peripheral resistance. There is actually very little movement of blood from the lower extremities back to the heart.

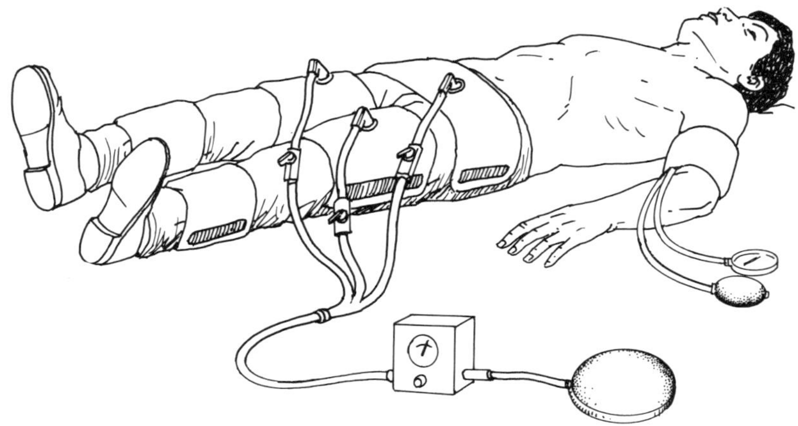

FIGURE 5.2 Pneumatic antishock garment.

The PASG is most useful in shock involving bleeding beneath the garmet (as, for example, in the case of pelvic fractures). Inflation of the PASG compresses the blood vessels and decreases bleeding (Figure 5.3). It also increases blood pressure. Although both of these effects are beneficial, studies have shown that PASG use does not appear to improve survival. In addition, there are a number of circumstances where PASG inflation may be harmful:

- bleeding outside the confines of the garment
- cardiogenic shock
- major chest injury
- ruptured hemidiaphragm
- evisceration
- pregnancy
- impalement

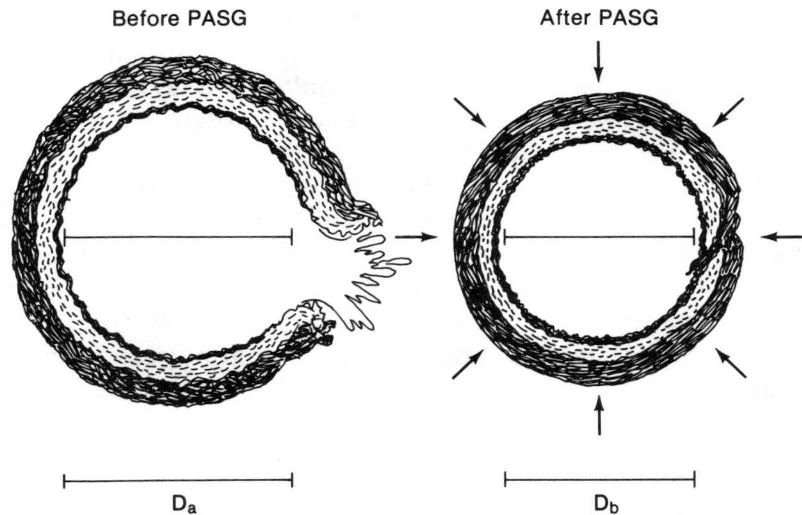

FIGURE 5.3 PASG inflation reduces vessel diameter (D) and slows bleeding.

Caution!
The PASG can compromise ventilation when the abdominal compartment is fully inflated. In the patient with respiratory distress, do not inflate the abdominal compartment unless directed by Medical Control.

Caution!
Use of the PASG is controversial. Know your local protocol and seek Medical Control if circumstances warrant.

TYPES OF SHOCK

Any process that interferes with adequate tissue perfusion can cause shock. In the trauma patient, shock is generally one of three types:

Hypovolemic Shock

This type of shock results from fluid volume deficit. Hemorrhagic hypovolemic shock, the type more frequently seen in traumatic settings, is due to the loss of blood or plasma. It can be caused by external losses, internal losses, burns, and crush injuries. Nonhemorrhagic hypovolemic shock results from dehydration due to sweating, vomiting, or diarrhea. The treatment is to stop the fluid loss, if possible, and to rapidly replace it.

Patients in hypovolemic shock need to be transported to a definitive care hospital as soon as possible. Some will require immediate surgery if they are to survive. In the field it is frequently impossible to determine which patients will need this type of care. But in all cases, establish an airway, administer oxygen, maintain normal temperature, minimize pain, and monitor the patient. Control external hemorrhage with pressure dressings and elevation. Avoid tourniquets except to prevent exsanguination. Look carefully for less obvious injuries. Raise the lower extremities or the lower end of the spine board—but, no more than 12 inches. You may apply the PASG and inflate it if protocol allows. Transport the patient promptly in an immobilized and supine position.

Cardiogenic Shock

Cardiogenic shock is due to failure of the pump (heart failure). Although cardiogenic shock commonly has nontraumatic causes (ischemia, infarct, valvular disease, severe arrhythmias, pulmonary embolism), it can also result from cardiac failure caused by cardiac tamponade and tension pneumothorax. The low cardiac output observed with these traumatic injuries is due to impaired filling of the heart. Patients in cardiogenic shock will often have difficulty breathing. Their pulse may be weak and irregular. Neck veins will usually be distended. Cardiac tamponade may cause muffling of heart sounds. In the patient with tension pneumothorax, breath sounds will usually be absent on one side and the trachea will be shifted to the opposite side. Cardiac contusion can also lead to heart failure and/or arrythmia, shock, and death.

Patients in cardiogenic shock should not have their legs elevated or the PASG applied. Give oxygen and reassurance and promptly transport them to the hospital.

Neurogenic Shock

Spinal cord injuries can cause loss of control of blood vessel tone and dilation of the vascular system. Blood then pools in the venous system and less blood returns to the heart. Low cardiac output follows, typically with no increase in heart rate. Often there is blood loss as well. With these patients, protect the spine at all times.

Institute general measures for neurogenic shock. Establish an airway, administer oxygen, maintain normal temperature, immobilize the spine, and monitor. Raise the foot of the spine board, but no more than 12 inches. Apply the PSAG according to local protocol.

CONCLUSION

In cases of shock, the most important action is to safely, efficiently, and rapidly transport the patient to the appropriate institution for definitive treatment. The general measures of improving oxygenation, stopping external blood loss, minimizing pain, and maintaining normal temperature will help prevent or diminish the consequences of shock.

Caution!
A patient in shock needs immediate definitive care, usually by a surgeon, not by an EMT. Do not be lulled into spending valuable time on the scene managing non-life-threatening wounds. Transport is the most important treatment for a patient in shock.

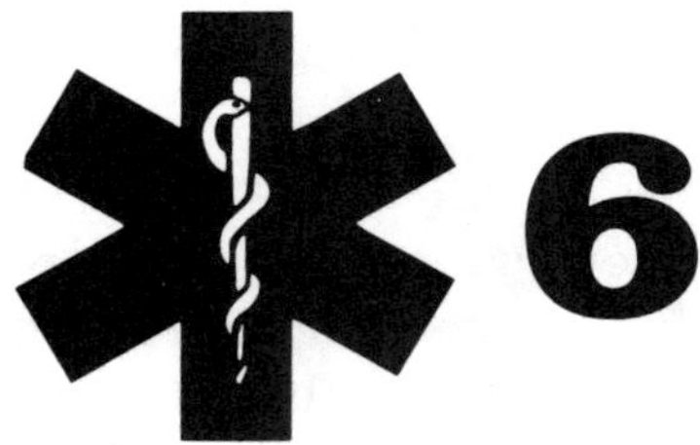

6

Head Injuries

INTRODUCTION

Head injury is the leading cause of death from blunt trauma. Over half of trauma-related deaths fall into this group, and the morbidity or impairment among the survivors is even more staggering. A large number of patients with survivable head injuries die from *secondary brain injury*. The leading causes of secondary brain injury are hypoxia and hypotension. Therefore, the first axiom of trauma care—Do No Further Harm—is important in dealing with the head-injured patient. Not only is death from secondary brain injury possible, but even mild brain injury can result in lasting deficits if hypotension or hypoxia persists. This chapter focuses on the recognition of head trauma, the understanding of the concept of progressive impairment, and the prevention of secondary brain injury.

OBJECTIVES

At the conclusion of this chapter, you should be able to:

1. Describe the basic anatomy and physiology of the brain.
2. Correlate certain clinical findings with their anatomic abnormalities and define urgency of care.
3. Distinguish among concussion, contusion, and hematoma and decide which require quick transport and operation and why.

ANATOMY AND FUNCTIONING OF THE BRAIN

A basic understanding of the normal anatomy and functioning of the brain allows one to appreciate the effects of certain injuries on brain function and body function. It then becomes obvious why there is such a high rate of mortality and morbidity associated with head injury.

The brain is a semisolid organ that constitutes about 2 percent of the body weight of an adult. It is composed of two cerebral hemispheres, the pons and the cerebellum, and the medulla oblongata (brain stem). The brain performs may functions. It mediates the functioning of the various systems of the body in order to maintain homeostasis. It controls the body and its very ability to exist as an organism. It is the seat of emotions, thought, and creativity. The brain is a very complicated organ and is very susceptible to dysfunction when injured. Brain injuries thus have dire consequences for the entire body.

The brain is well protected by the skull, or cranium (Figure 6.1). The adult skull is rigid, and composed of immovable fused bones. The skull is protected by the scalp—a highly vascular multilayer structure covered by skin.

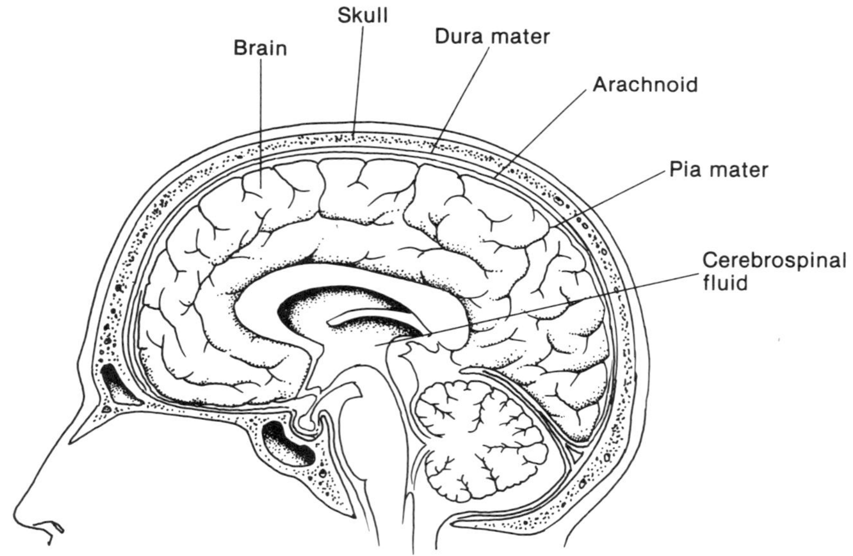

FIGURE 6.1 Sagittal section of the head.

The brain is further protected by three coverings called meninges (Figure 6.2). These layers protect and suspend the brain within the skull. The outer layer is known as the dura mater, and is composed of strong fibrous tissue. It also serves as the periosteum for the skull. The arachnoid is the middle layer. The pia mater is the innermost layer and overlays the brain surface.

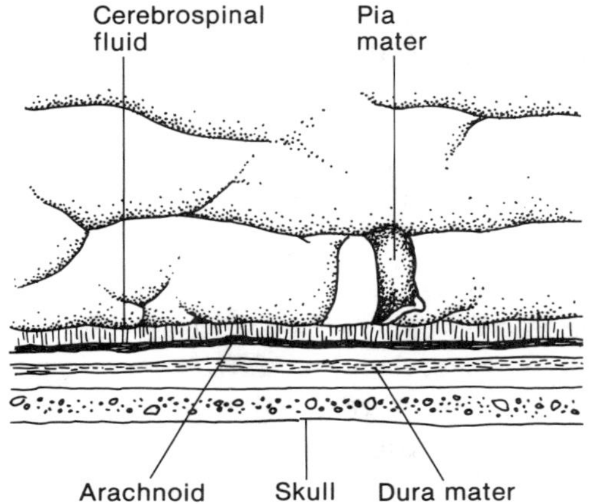

FIGURE 6.2 The meninges.

The brain has a higher oxygen requirement than the rest of the body. Although it constitues only 2 percent of body weight, it utilizes approximately 20 percent of the body's oxygen. This is a crucial requirement, since the brain cannot store energy and thus cannot survive even temporarily through anaerobic metabolism, as can skeletal muscle and other tissues. An interruption of oxygenated blood for more than four minutes almost always results in brain damage. Blood reaches the brain through the internal carotid arteries and the vertebral arteries. The internal jugular veins carry the majority of blood away from the brain, ending in the superior vena cava.

TYPES OF HEAD INJURIES

Scalp Lacerations

The most common form of head injury is a scalp laceration. Scalp lacerations are caused by the head striking some object, such as a car windshield, or by some object striking the head. The scalp is very vascular and bleeds profusely if the laceration is large. Shock can set in if the bleeding is not controlled quickly.

Most scalp lacerations are best managed in the field by the application of a sterile dressing and compression bandage. Avulsion is a type of scalp laceration resulting in partial separation of a flap of tissue. Although much more serious in appearance and more significant in terms of blood loss, it can be treated returning the flap to its normal position and covering the area with a sterile dressing and a compression bandage. Avulsions often require ingenuity to bandage, for the proper bandage depends on size and location of the wound.

Skull Fractures

These are the second most common form of head injury. There may be little external evidence of a fracture. If there is no laceration to the scalp, the fracture is considered a *closed fracture.* Some lacerations or fractures extend into the paranasal sinuses or the middle ear, resulting in cerebrospinal fluid leak. These fractures are regarded as *open fractures.*

Like long-bone fractures, skull fractures may be categorized as linear, comminuted, or depressed. *Linear fractures* are by far the most common and are frequently diagnosed only by X-ray. Approximately half of all linear skull fractures involve the temporal and parietal bones of the skull.

The compound fracture, a form of open fracture, is more serious. It may present as a small laceration above a skull fracture, or it may involve a very grotesque injury with exposed skull fragments and possibly exposed brain tissue. Always consider such an injury serious, and manage it with careful application of sterile dressings. The bandage should tamponade bleeding but not be so tight as to force bone fragments into the brain.

The third type of skull fracture is the *depressed fracture.* It may be present in the absence of a laceration. A depressed skull fracture is suggested by an area of depression of the skull, but often there is no external evidence. Damage to the underlying brain may co-exist.

Depending on the location of the skull fracture, various signs and symptoms may be present. These include Battle's signs (bruising behind the ear), raccoon eyes (Figure 6.3), and blood or cerebrospinal fluid leakage from the ears or nose.

Patients with head injury may also suffer injuries to the brain

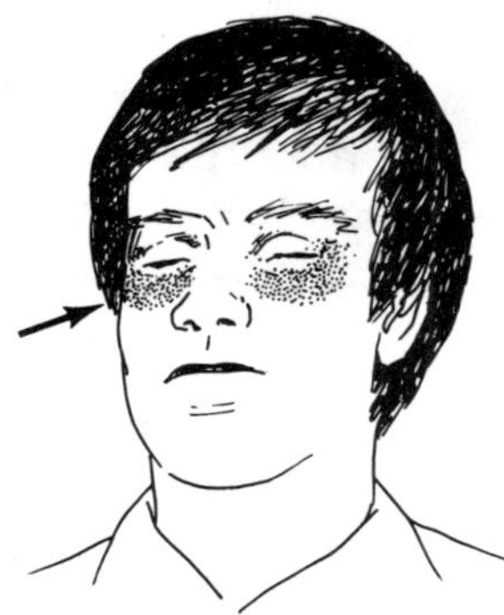

FIGURE 6.3 Raccoon eyes in patient with depressed skull fracture.

itself, which are known as intracranial injuries. The most common cause of intracranial injury is motor vehicle accidents. Other significant causes are gunshot wounds and blunt trauma from falls, athletic injuries, or contact by an object.

Closed Head Injury

Blunt injury to the brain is referred to as closed head injury. Such injuries are of several types.

Concussion. This injury may be mild or moderate. The victim of a mild concussion suffers a brief diminution in level of consciousness. The resulting confusion or disorientation clears spontaneously after a few minutes. The victim may be unable to recall the circumstances of the accident or what occurred either immediately before or after the accident. Witnesses to the accident may provide clues to the presence of a concussion.

A moderate concussion is one resulting in a loss of consciousness of more than a few minutes but less than 24 hours. This patient is unconscious at the scene, but will generally recover in the hospital with a minimum of definitive care. Rarely will there be significant neurological defects, although there may be minor personality changes or memory loss. A common statement by friends or family is that the victim somehow is "different than he was before the accident." Concussions are characterized pathologically by an absence of anatomic brain injury.

Contusion. This is a more serious form of closed head injury. Permanent defects are common. The degree of functional impairment depends on the damage to the individual areas of the brain.

Severe Contusion (diffuse brain injury). Here the patient is immediately rendered unconscious by the trauma and remains so for a long period. The patient is often left permanently impaired. This type of injury may be immediately detectable at the scene in the form of disruptions in normal respiratory and vital-sign patterns.

Hematomas. Concussion, contusion, and diffuse brain injury are quite common. Less common but of greater importance from a treatment standpoint are hematomas. Three types will be briefly described: subdural, epidural, and intracrainial.

Subdural hematoma (SDH). This is the most common form of hematoma. It is caused by bleeding into the potential space between the dura mater and the arachnoid. Subdural bleeding may be classified as either acute or chronic. Acute subdural hematoma occurs within 72 hours of the head injury. The seriousness of the hematoma depends on its size and on how fast it collects. Subdural hematoma often carries a high mortality rate especially if it develops early and rapidly after the injury. The only definitive treatment for an expanding subdural hematoma is surgical evacuation of the blood or clot. A subdural hematoma cannot be diagnosed on the scene, but a change in level of consciousness or changes in pupil reaction and motor responses commonly follow it (Figure 6.4).

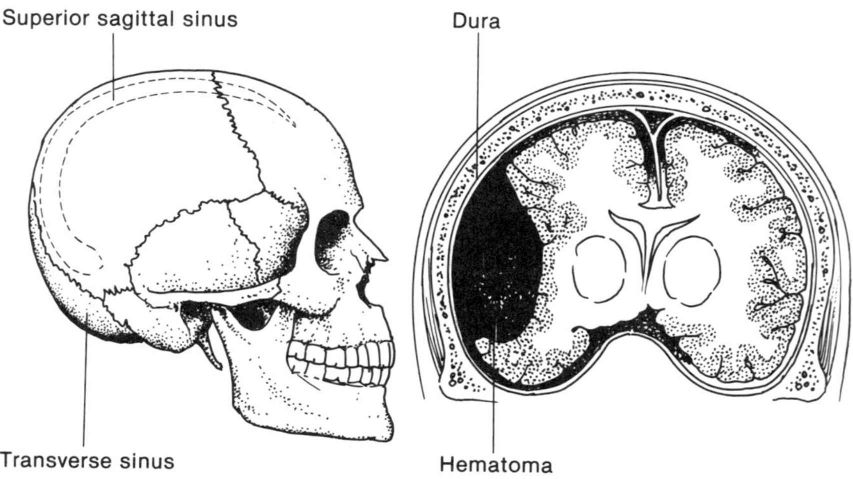

FIGURE 6.4 Subdural hematoma.

Epidural hematoma. This is caused by laceration of the middle meningeal artery, which in turn often results from fracture of the temporal bone (Figure 6.5). Indeed, any laceration or detectable skull fracture above and forward of the ear in the region of the temple is potentially serious. A patient may initially be alert and oriented and then become disoriented or even unconscious (Figure 6.6). It is important that epidural hematomas be suspected

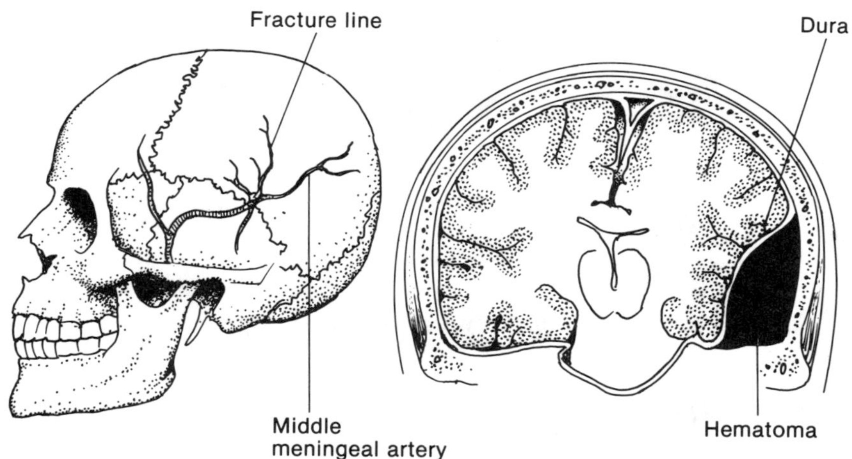

FIGURE 6.5 Epidural hematoma.

in any patient who has suffered a head injury. Mortality is lower for patients with epidural hematoma than for patients with subdural hematoma, but treatment must be prompt.

Intracranial hematoma. Also known as subarachnoid hemorrhage, this hematoma occurs in the potential space between the arachnoid layer and the brain itself. Subarachnoid hemorrhage is less common than other types of bleeding but is still serious.

Intracranial bleeding has various effects on the brain, which in turn affect the entire body. Generally these effects are progressive as the bleeding continues.

Patients with head injuries must be constantly reevaluated. Conduct your evaluation the same way each time and note any changes. Never leave a patient with a head injury alone at an accident scene—neurological deterioration can occur rapidly.

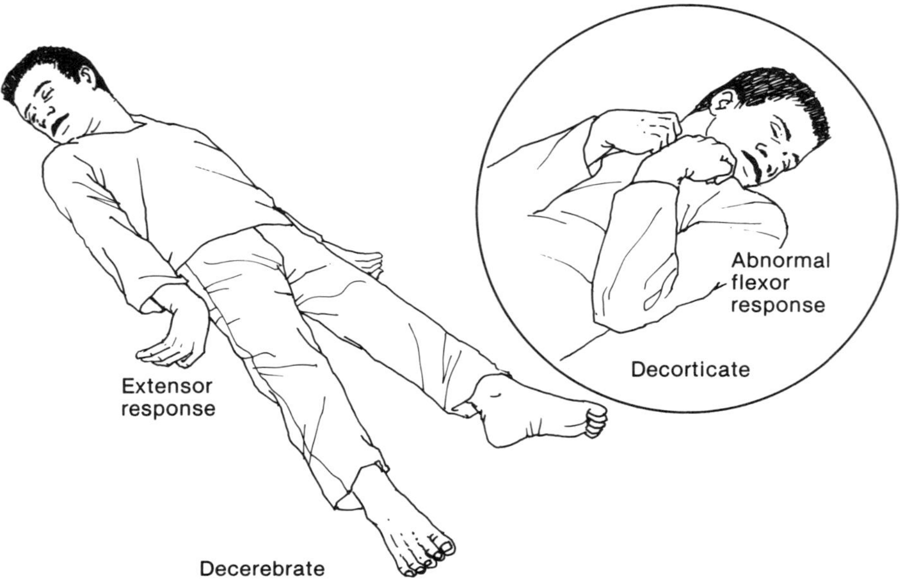

FIGURE 6.6 Two types of posturing.

ASSESSMENT

Begins by evaluating the information in the dispatch call, and continue your assessment as you arrive at the scene. A brief overview of the scene is in order, which should take no more than 15 to 20 seconds. Note the positions of the crashed vehicles; they may give you an idea of how the crash occurred. Observing the damage to both the outside and the inside should give you further clues as to how the occupant(s) may have been injured. Such obvious things as whether or not the victim was wearing a seat belt and shoulder harness should be immediately noted. Is the windshield damaged from inside? Is there blood on the windshield? Is the steering wheel damaged? All of these may indicate that the driver struck his head on the inside of the car. This phase of assessment should be brief and done as the victim is approached. Although this discussion has focused on an automobile crash, the EMT should always consider the mechanisms of injury during any incident involving head or other types of injuries.

Quite often you must rely on others for a history of the event. Bystanders can be both helpful and frustrating. Some experienced EMTs refuse to listen to bystanders who try to tell them what happened, or they tune them out as they go about patient assessment and treatment. But in the case of a head-injury victim, a bystander may be the only source of information other than what you can observe at the incident scene. If circumstances allow, you can obtain a history from bystanders while your partner assesses the patient. Some of the information may not be reliable. For example, time is often difficult to measure during a crisis. A bystander may tell you the victim was unconscious for 10 or 15 minutes when in fact he was unconscious only 2 minutes. The important fact to note is that the victim was unconscious—a possible indication of a concussion. On the other hand, a bystander may tell you a victim who was found unconscious some distance from his vehicle had gotten out of the wrecked car, walked around, and even looked at the damage before sitting down on the curb and lapsing into unconsciousness. This is very pertinent.

Begin your definitive assessment as you approach the victim. Is he moving? Is he breathing? If so, are his respirations rapid or slow, even or labored? Is there any external hemorrhage? Is the victim conscious? What is his skin color?

The most important assessment item is the victim's level of consciousness. Several methods have been developed to assess and monitor level of consciousness. Among these are the AVPU system and the Glasgow Coma Scale. Use both in your evaluation of the victim.

The AVPU system characterizes the victim according to her best responses. *A* refers to *alert.* The victim is completely alert and conversing. She requires no external stimuli to awaken her. *V* refers to *voice.* The victim will awaken to a voice or will move her extremities in response to a voice command. *P* stands for *pain* or painful stimuli. The victim is not alert and will not respond to a voice, but will move her arms or legs in response to the application of a painful stimulus such as a pinch. It is important to note whether the responses are appropriate or inappropriate. Does she move her arm away from the pinch, or does she use the opposite hand to remove the pinch? Any movement to remove the noxious stimulus is purposeful and appropriate. Does she extend her arm and leg on one side or both sides? Such responses are not appropriate and indicate severe head injury. *U,* the last and most serious category, indicates that the victim is *unresponsive;* she does not respond to any type of stimuli, verbal or painful. Such a system may be useful in the triage of multiple victims when incorporated into an evaluation of other injuries. If a painful stimulus is applied, record the types of stimulus used so later examiners can determine any change.

> **Caution!**
> When applying a painful stimulus, use the AVPU method and document fully the stimulus, how it was applied, and the response. Trends can be determined only by accurate information.

The Glasgow Coma Scale (Table 6.1) allows you to evaluate three criteria: eye opening, best verbal response, and best motor response. The victim is scored first on what type of stimulus is required to make him open his eyes. According to the scale, the victim who opens his eyes spontaneously receives a score of 4 for eye opening. (Note that this does not apply to the comatose patient whose eyes are open constantly.) A victim who opens his eyes to a painful stimulus applied to an extremity would receive only a 2. The patient who does not open his eyes is given only one point.

Table 6.1
Glasgow Coma Scale (GCS)

Add scores for eye opening, best verbal response, and best motor response.

Eye opening	Best verbal response	Best motor response
Spontaneous = 4	Oriented = 5	Obeys commands = 6
To voice = 3	Confused = 4	Localizes pain = 5
To pain = 2	Inappropriate words = 3	Withdraws to pain = 4
None = 1	Incomprehensible sounds = 2	Flexion to pain = 3
	None = 1	Extension to pain = 2
		None = 1
		Total Score:

Assessment of best verbal response is scored similarly. If the patient is alert and oriented as to (person, place, and time), she receives a score of 5. At the opposite end of the scale, the patient who does not speak receives a 1.

In the evaluation of best motor response, a patient who obeys commands receives a score of 6. The best performance by any extremity is the appropriate one for scoring. If the patient localizes a painful stimulus and tries to remove it, the score is 5. Withdrawal from the painful stimulus warrants 4 points. Posturing (Figure 6.6) indicates more severe brain injury. If the arms are flexed (decorticate posturing), give a score of 3. If the patient extends his extremities (decerebrate posturing), give a score of 2. If there is no response to pain the victim receives a score of 1. This may indicate a very serious brain injury or possibly a spinal cord injury.

You may not have time to write down the Glasgow Coma Scale score during your initial evaluation and assessment of the patient. In fact, that is not recommended. The AVPU system is more appropriate for an initial field assessment of level of consciousness. The Glasgow Coma Scale, properly utilized, is valuable for evaluating changes in level of consciousness, especially during a long transport. The three parameters of eye opening, best verbal response, and best motor response should be reassessed periodically along with vital signs.

Next, assess the pupils as part of the initial neurological examination. In the alert patient, pupils of unequal size should not be regarded as a bad sign. Remember that a certain proportion of the population has this characteristic. Also, certain medications and recreational drugs have an effect on pupil size and reaction. Don't be confused by evidence of previous eye surgery or the presence of a glass eye.

Caution!
Level of consciousness is the best indicator of overall neurological function. Reassess it frequently in the field.

MANAGEMENT

The first step is to check for a patent airway. Airway patency is the most important measure in assessing and treating a victim of traumatic head injury. The importance of a patent airway cannot be overemphasized. In an alert, communicative patient who exhibits no respiratory distress, the airway is not a problem. In the unresponsive patient, the establishment of a patent airway may be a great problem. The incidence of cervical spine injury in the head-injured patient is approximately 5 percent. Unstable spine fractures are less likely, but because of the possibility of a cervical spine injury, you should establish the airway by using a jaw thrust. Grasp the angle of the mandible on either side of the face with both hands and pull forward slightly while maintaining the cervical spine in neutral position. This action opens the airway by displacing the tongue forward. The neck lift is no longer recommended as a method to open the airway. You can now check for blood, teeth, vomitus, or foreign matter in the upper airway. In the absence of a gag reflex, you may want to insert an oropharyngeal airway. But remember, such an airway will not be tolerated by a conscious or semiconscious patient. Stimulation of the gag reflex may cause the victim to become restless or combative or may cause vomiting, which may block the airway and lead to an aspiration pneumonia.

Next, reassess the adequacy of respirations. Upon opening the airway, you can quickly assess the color of the mucous membranes. Listening for breath sounds may not be reliable at a noisy accident scene or in the back of the ambulance. If ventilation is inadequate, help the victim breathe by using a demand valve or a bag-valve-mask (you will need a partner for this) with 100 percent oxygen. Even if ventilation is adequate, always administer supplementary oxygen. In the fully alert victim, you can do this with a nasal cannula. In the semiconscious or completely unconscious victim, use a nonrebreathing mask with 100 percent oxygen. Check constantly for vomiting. This is especially important if the victim has a tight-fitting oxygen mask over his face, because any vomitus will be forced back into the upper airway.

The next assessment priority is to verify that the patient has adequate circulation. While establishing the airway and administering supplementary oxygen, check for a strong, regular carotid pulse. Is the pulse extremely slow with strong bounding? Is the carotid weak and thready and very rapid? The former may indicate increased intracranial pressure; the latter may indicate hypovolemia (in which case you may use a PASG, local protocol permitting).

Caution!
Your most important job is to protect the patient from secondary brain injury—avoid hypoxia and hypotension.

If the patient has an airway and is receiving oxygen, the most urgent priority is to reestablish cerebral-tissue perfusion. To do you must restore blood pressure. Cerebral perfusion pressure (CPP) is the pressure needed to assure adequate cerebral circulation. Intracerebral pressure (ICP) is the pressure within the confines of the skull. In considering the possibility of secondary brain injury, remember this equation:

$$CPP = BP - ICP$$

Clearly, a low BP and a high ICP can critically reduce CPP, causing brain ischemia.

At this point, apply a cervical collar and reassess airway integrity. Check for fractures. Control serious bleeding with pressure dressings. Splint major long-bone fractures before moving the victim, unless there is serious airway or respiratory inadequacy that cannot be corrected on the scene. In this case, strap the patient to a long spine board and transport as quickly as possible. You can immobilize fractures and bandage wounds during transport as long as you remember to maintain the airway and assist ventilation. Always consider the first priorities of airway, ventilation, and shock management in dealing with head-injury victims, even if they have other serious injuries.

TRANSPORT

The transport phase is critical to survival of the patient. Transport should be rapid but not reckless. If you are in the back of the ambulance assisting ventilation, the ride must be stable enough for you to do so effectively.

Transport the patient to the closest appropriate facility. This usually means a trauma center. If there is no trauma center locally, then transport the patient to the hospital most capable of dealing with the patient's head injuries. The patient may be alert enough to choose a hospital. Or a family member on the scene may do this. Be aware that such a preference may not be the most appropriate for the patient. If there is disagreement on this issue, contact Medical Control. Depending on local protocol, the injured patient may be transported to the hospital of her choice.

During transport, continually reassess the patient. Reevaluate airway, respiratory adequacy, circulatory status, and level of consciousness at frequent intervals. Constantly observe the patient. A good secondary survey may locate previously undetected injuries. You can complete your run report at the hospital.

Make a patient report to the receiving hospital as soon as possible after transport has begun. Call in any pertinent change in the victim's status. If caring for the victim prevents you from talking on the radio, the driver should handle radio communications. Teamwork and communication with your EMT team is essential.

CONCLUSION

Head injuries are common but complicated. Yet field management is simple. Even if injury is significant, the priority of care is the same. Establish and maintain the airway. Ensure adequate respirations. Oxygen is a must. Verify circulation in the form of a strong carotid pulse, and fully immobilize the patient on a spine board. Perform a good neurological examination and repeat during transport. Transport the victim to a trauma center, if available. Frequently communicate patient status to the receiving institution.

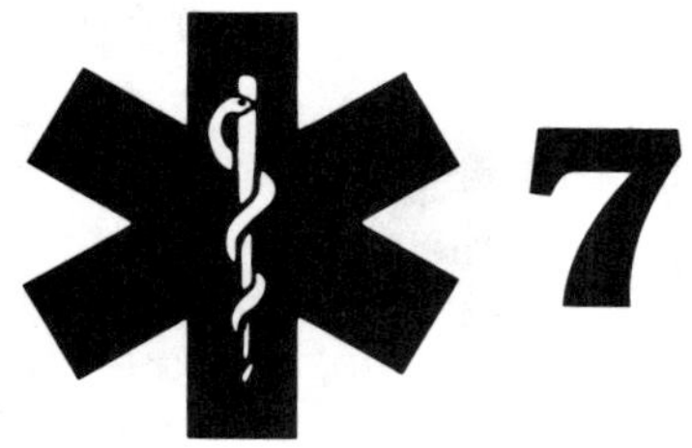

7

Spine and Spinal Cord Injury

INTRODUCTION

Injuries to the spine and spinal cord are common and often devastating. The acute onset of the injury combined with the immediate implications for long-term impairment cause profound anxiety in patients who suddenly cannot move their legs. Spinal immobilization is an oft-practiced skill. Head injured patients are at increased risk for spine or spinal cord injuries. One in ten multiple-trauma patients sustain some sort of spinal injury. Male victims of automobile accidents between 18 and 35 years of age are most commonly affected. In the U.S., it is estimated that the average annual rate of spinal trauma is about 50 persons per million population, and half of these victims die within a year of their injury.

EMTs have an important role in the management of the spinal-injured patient. The initial management rendered at the scene may determine whether these patients regain normal function or are disabled for life. Preventing further injury while in transport to the hospital is paramount. The key to prevention is thinking about the possibility of spinal injury before the patient is moved. Improper field management of spinal-injured patients can be catastrophic. Fortunately, techniques for managing this type of patient are easy to learn and follow. The spine board, cervical collar, and cervical immobilization device (CID) are familiar pieces of equipment to the EMT.

OBJECTIVES

At the completion of this chapter, you should be able to:

1. Explain the importance of spinal trauma, its potential for causing lifelong impairment, and why prevention of further injury is important.
2. Correlate the anatomy of the bony elements of the spine with the anatomy of the spinal cord and the common mechanisms of injury.
3. Define the function of the spinal cord and the changes found with injury at various levels.
4. Recognize which patients are at risk for spinal trauma and by what mechanism.
5. Describe a neurologic examination and define what changes are expected with cervical, thoracic, and lumbar injuries.
6. List the devices used in the immobilization of the spine and their proper application.

ANATOMY OF THE SPINE

The spine is a collection of bones joined together by joints. It serves as the main structure for axial support of the body. The spinal cord, contained within the spine, is part of the central nervous system. Understanding the anatomic relationship of the spinal column to the spinal cord is important in preventing further injury.

The spinal column is made up of bones or vertebrae that are divided into five anatomical segments (Figure 7.1). The bones of each segment vary slightly from those of other segments but have similar functions: to serve as structural support for the body, and to protect the spinal cord.

The five types of bones in the spinal column are as follows:

1. The cervical vertebrae: These consist of the first seven bones of the neck. They are numbered C1 through C7, C1 being the first vertebra of the spinal column. It is easy to feel C7; it's the large, hard knot you can feel at the base of your neck if you bend your head forward.
2. The thoracic bones: These are the next 12 vertebra. They are called *thoracic* because they define the chest cavity, or thorax. They are numbered T1 through T12. Each thoracic vertebra is attached to a pair of ribs.

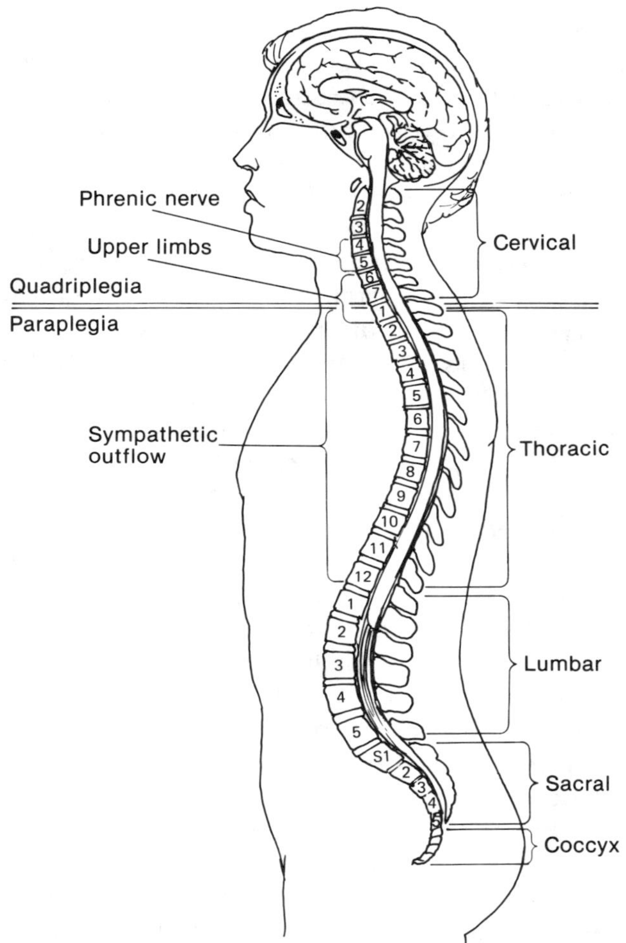

FIGURE 7.1 Normal spinal column and anatomic segments.

3. The lumbar vertebrae: These are the largest of all. They consist of the five bones of the lower back and are numbered L1 through L5.
4. The sacrum: This appears to be one large bone but is actually five separate vertebra that are fused together. The sacrum is part of the pelvis.
5. The coccyx (tailbone): This is actually three to four fused bones appearing as one. The coccyx is also commonly considered part of the pelvis.

Each vertebra consists of a solid body, or anterior portion, and a vertebral arch, or posterior portion. The vertebral bodies are the weight-bearing portions of the spine. Because of this they are the most commonly injured part of the spinal column. Through the vertebral arch passes the spinal cord and spinal nerve roots. While these areas are much less likely to be injured (because they are well protected by the spinal bodies and the muscles that surround them), injuries to these areas are responsible for most of the damage to the spinal cord. Each vertebra is separated from the next by a disc that serves as a cushion and allows motion in the spine.

The spinal cord is actually a continuation of the brain outside of the skull, and it has many functions. Its primary function is to carry electrical messages from the brain to the rest of the body and back again (Figure 7.2). It also serves as the reflex arc center of the nervous system. This nerve cable extends down through the center of the vertebral arch, or foramen, with nerve branches exiting between every pair of vertebra. The spinal cord itself ends at the level of the first or second lumbar vertebra, but smaller nerve fibers—the corda equina—extend down to the sacrum. Any injury to the spinal cord will impair its ability to carry vital electrical messages to and from the brain. Whether a bruise, pressure exerted from a neighboring structure, or a partial or complete tear of the cord itself, an injury to the spinal cord is very serious.

Respiration is controlled by the phrenic nerve. The roots of this nerve leave the cervical spine at the fourth and fifth intervertebral spaces. Transection of the cord above this level will cause respiratory arrest and possibly death. Injuries below the level of C5 but above the thoracic vertebrae will cause the patient to breathe with the diaphragm only. The effects of transection of the spinal cord are dramatic. All motor, sensory, and reflex activity below the level of transection is lost. Fracture or dislocation of the spinal column without damage to the spinal cord is possible, but the potential for injury is always present. It is also possible for damage of the spinal cord to occur without damage to the bones of the spine. It is best to assume that all trauma patients, even if seemingly uninjured at first, have spinal injury. Because of this, all trauma patients must be handled and packaged for transport in such a way that their entire spinal column is protected from further injury.

The cervical spine is the most commonly injured part of the spinal column. Because of the cervical spine's proximity to the

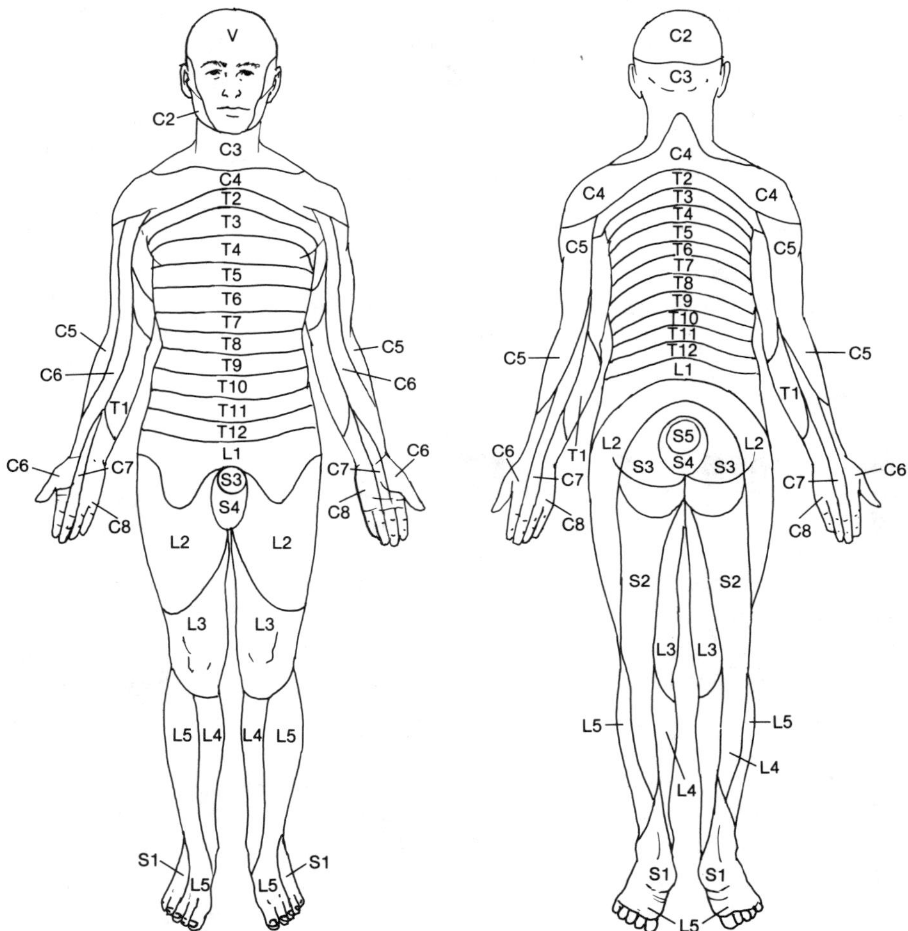

FIGURE 7.2 Areas of the body controlled by various levels of the spinal cord.

skull, any injury to the head will transmit force downward to it. Therefore, any patient with a head injury is at increased risk for fracture dislocation of the cervical spine and associated injury to the spinal cord. Automobile crashes are a primary cause of this injury.

The thoracic spine is much better protected by surrounding structures than the cervical spine. The muscles of the back, ribs, and chest all serve to protect the thoracic spine. However, the intervertebral foramina of the thoracic spine are smaller than those in the rest of the spinal column. Because of this, injuries to the thoracic spine will likely involve damage to the spinal cord.

The most common injury to the lumbar spine is a compression fracture of the vertebral body. Because the spinal cord ends above the lumbosacral region, and because the posterior portions of the lumbar spine are well protected, spinal cord injury resulting from lumbar injuries is less frequent.

Caution!
Injury to the spinal column at one level means a greater risk of coexisting injury at another level.

MECHANISM OF INJURY

Spinal injury is more likely in certain situations:

Motor Vehicle Crashes. This is the most common cause of spinal trauma. Practically every type of spinal injury can occur in a motor vehicle crash. Victims who are ejected are particularly vulnerable. *All* crash victims must be assumed to have spinal injuries and should be treated accordingly.

Falls. Any fall can cause a spinal injury. Striking the head against the ground or an object can cause significant strain upon the neck. Falling from a great height and landing on the feet will likely cause a compression fracture in either the thoracic or lumbar spine. Observe and report the circumstances surrounding any fall injury.

Sports. Almost any physical sport can cause spinal injuries. Most fatal football injuries are caused by cervical spine fractures. Boxing, wrestling, and other contact sports, gymnastics, biking, and skiing may produce spinal injuries.

Diving. Units often respond to a drowning call to find the victim has hit his head while diving into water. Hitting the head while diving can injure the neck. These patients should be removed from the water on a long spine board and have a cervical collar applied.

Electrocution. Aside from causing a fall or throwing the victim against a solid object, electric shock may cause strong muscle spasms. The spine may be injured in any of these ways.

Penetrating Trauma. Gunshot and knife wounds to the head, neck, or trunk can damage the spine and spinal cord. Direct laceration of the cord is possible.

TYPES OF INJURIES

Cervical Strain. Cervical strain—or whiplash, as it is commonly called—is a hyperextension injury in which the head snaps backward. It occurs most commonly in motor vehicle crashes where the auto is hit from behind. If the vehicle lacks a properly fitted headrest, head will travel through a greater arc, damaging the ligaments and muscles of the neck (see Chapter 1).

Wedge Fracture. This is usually a hyperflexion injury caused by vertical loading with the spine in the flexed position. It is seen in the cervical, thoracic, and lumbar vertebrae.

Compression Fracture. Downward force applied to the spine may cause a crushing of the body, or anterior portion, of the vertebra. Compression fractures are common in falls where the victim lands on the feet. It is not uncommon to find fractures of the calcaneus, or heel bone, along with this injury.

Central Cord Syndrome. This unusual problem occurs when only part of the spinal cord is damaged. Only the arms of the patient are affected, even though the injury to the cord may be in the neck. You will not be able to make this diagnosis in the field. Always record the neurological status of all trauma patients before and after placing them on spine boards and before and after any manipulation of their neck.

Neurogenic Shock. This condition is caused by loss of the sympathetic control of the peripheral circulation, leading to profound vasodilation. This causes pooling of blood in the skin and extremities. People in neurogenic shock have a lowered blood pressure that may confuse their condition with hypovolemic shock, especially in the trauma patient. Although the patient's blood pressure may indicate shock, the patient does not appear pale, does not have moist, sweaty skin, and usually has a normal pulse rate.

> **Caution!**
> The person in neurogenic shock may also be bleeding.

MANAGEMENT

Techniques

When responding to any call for assistance the first step is to review the dispatch information. Always try to think ahead. At the scene, look over the accident site carefully, and try to avoid "tunnel vision." Observe and note anything that might lead you to suspect back or neck trauma.

Neurologic Exam. This is part of the secondary survey, although you can gain much information when you first approach the patient. If the patient appears alert, is conversing, and seems to be moving all extremities, then much of the neurological exam is already done. First, ask the conscious patient if he is having any pain. Be alert to any indication of neck or back pain or any pain down either or both arms or legs. Tingling or numbness is noteworthy. Many patients will say that their arms and legs are numb or that they cannot move their extremities. But remember that the nonspecialist's definition of *numb* is often different from the examiner's. It is important to weed out false complaints during your assessment. Since pain and tingling are subjective complaints, be careful in your questioning. Always record the response to touch in all extremities before and after moving the patient. Record the patient's ability to move all extremities. Repeat this examination several times prior to and during transport to the hospital. If there is loss of sensation, record the level at which sensation stops. It is a good idea to make a mark on the skin of the abdomen or chest with a ball-point pen. Accurate documentation is mandatory for proper emergency medical care.

Any patient rendered unconscious following trauma must be assumed to have spinal injuries. The same is true for the injured person under the influence of alcohol or other drugs. Although the unconscious patient will probably not respond to commands, note and document any extremity movement.

Helmet Removal. Motorcyclists and participants in certain sports, especially football, are at a greater risk for injuries that may result in cervical spine trauma. Helmet use is common in many of these sports. In general, the helmet should be left in place unless it interferes with airway management or breathing. The patient can be immobilized with the helmet in place and transported safely. If the helmet requires removal in the field, one rescuer should immobilize the neck from below while the second rescuer removes the helmet from above (Figure 7.3).

Tools

Cervical Collar. The cervical collar is the first line of defense in the management of spinal injuries. It reminds the patient not to move the neck. It also helps maintain the cervical spine in a neutral position, thereby reducing the possibility of aggravating an existing cervical injury. There are many type of cervical collars. Although some are better at immobilization than others, none is totally protective. Some cervical collars are one-piece, and some come in two pieces. Many EMTs prefer the two-piece collar because they can briefly remove the front section to assess the patient's anterior neck. All cervical collars must be rigid enough to support the head while keeping the neck in neutral position. Soft collars are unacceptable.

Cervical Immobilization Device (CID). This consists of two padded foam blocks that fasten to a firm base, usually with Velcro. The base of the CID is placed at the head end of the spine board before the patient is placed on the board. After proper placement of the patient upon the spineboard, the padded blocks are attached on either side of the patient's head. Then two straps, one placed across the chin, one across the forehead, are fastened to the CID. This, in combination with a cervical collar, usually does an adequate job of immobilizing the patient's neck.

Long Spine Board. These are usually made out of wood. They are 72 inches long and come in varying widths. Most have hand

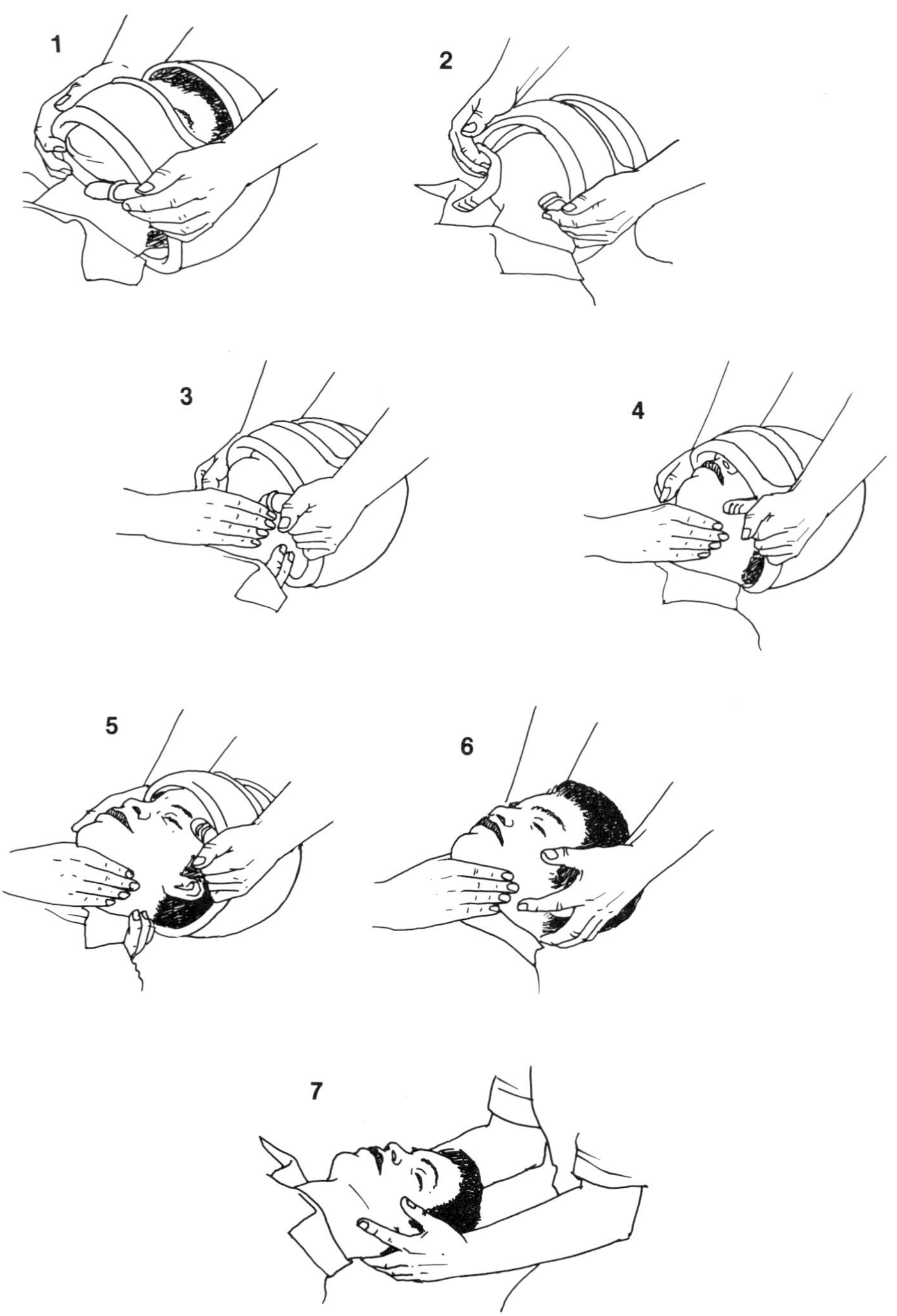

FIGURE 7.3 Proper technique for removing motorcycle helmet.

holes cut out along the perimeter. Some have runners along the bottom to allow the boards to be lifted easily from the ground. Similar to the long board is the folding aluminum board, which folds in the middle for easy storage in the ambulance. Another variation is the scoop stretcher. This device is also made from aluminum. It has tubular construction and separates by means of hinges in the middle of the long axis. The support is provided by thin metal shelves projecting from either side, not quite joining in the middle. The device is first separated and then placed on either side of the patient. Then the two sides are passed under the patient and reconnected at each end. The patient is literally scooped up from the ground. The length of the scoop stretcher may be varied, which contributes to its usefulness.

Caution!
The scoop stretcher does not provide adequate support to the back and neck. Take added care to protect the spine whenever a regular spine board cannot be used.

The patient must be strapped to the board. A minimum of three straps are recommended, across the knees, the pelvic area, and the chest. All efforts at immobilization are lost if the patient is spilled from the board during transport due to lack of proper strapping. Also, spinal-injured patients may vomit. Proper use of straps and the CID will allow you to raise the spine board to one side in the event of vomiting, thereby protecting the patient's airway and spine at the same time.

Short Spine Board. This is an extrication device, used primarily for an unconscious patient who is slumped over the dash in a vehicle. This device has lost favor among most EMTs because of its complicated application requirements. Variations with greater flexibility have been marketed and are better suited for confined spaces. Most substitutes for the standard short spine board require a special type of cervical collar. They all operate on the same principle. The board is slipped behind the patient while one EMT is immobilizing the patient's neck. After placing the board behind the patient, straps are fastened across the chest and around the thighs. The patient is then removed from the vehicle and placed onto a long spine board.

The short board does not support the thoracic or lumbar spine. Despite its complexity, it is a useful device for front- or rear-seat extrication. A long spine board is required when this device is used.

CONCLUSION

The key to proper management of spine and spinal cord injuries is to consider all injured patients at risk. Be alert to the mechanism of injury. Provide good, aggressive management with emphasis on the basic skills of immobilization. Provide gentle emergency care to these patients and when in doubt, immobilize.

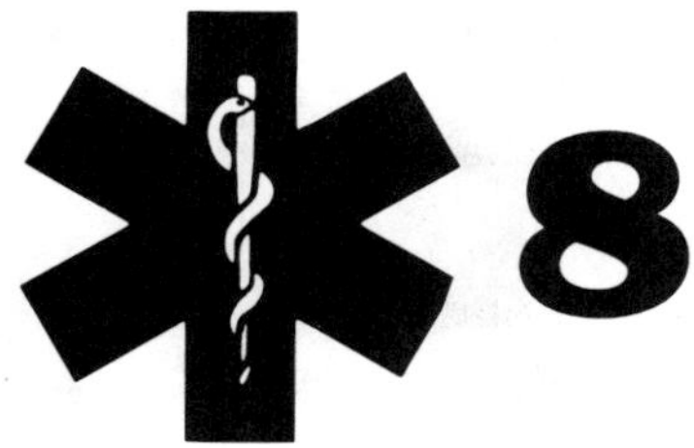

Abdominal Injuries

INTRODUCTION

Persons receiving high-energy forces to the abdomen (blunt or penetrating) are commonly encountered in the field. Abdominal trauma accounts for approximately 10 percent of deaths following blunt trauma. This is a significant percentage when you consider that the majority of deaths are preventable with prompt definitive surgical treatment.

You are at a disadvantage in dealing with victims of abdominal trauma, since there is very little you can do in the field. But your responsibility is great, because adbdominal trauma is such a time-sensitive problem. Undue delay in transport will harm the patient with internal bleeding, by prolonging the period of shock, increasing the need for blood transfusions, or contributing to prehospital trauma arrest. The challenge to the EMT is to recognize abdominal injury.

OBJECTIVES

At the completion of this chapter, you should be able to:

1. Define the two basic types of abdominal injuries and their risks to the patients.

2. Describe hollow and solid organs, give examples of each, and identify their functions.
3. List the anatomic divisions of the abdomen and the organs each contains, and explain the clinical significance of symptons by quadrants.
4. Describe signs and symptoms of abdominal trauma evident from the history of the accident and inspection and palpation of the abdomen.
5. Explain how physical findings may help distinguish between hollow-organ and solid-organ injuries.
6. State the principles of field care of patients with suspected abdominal trauma.

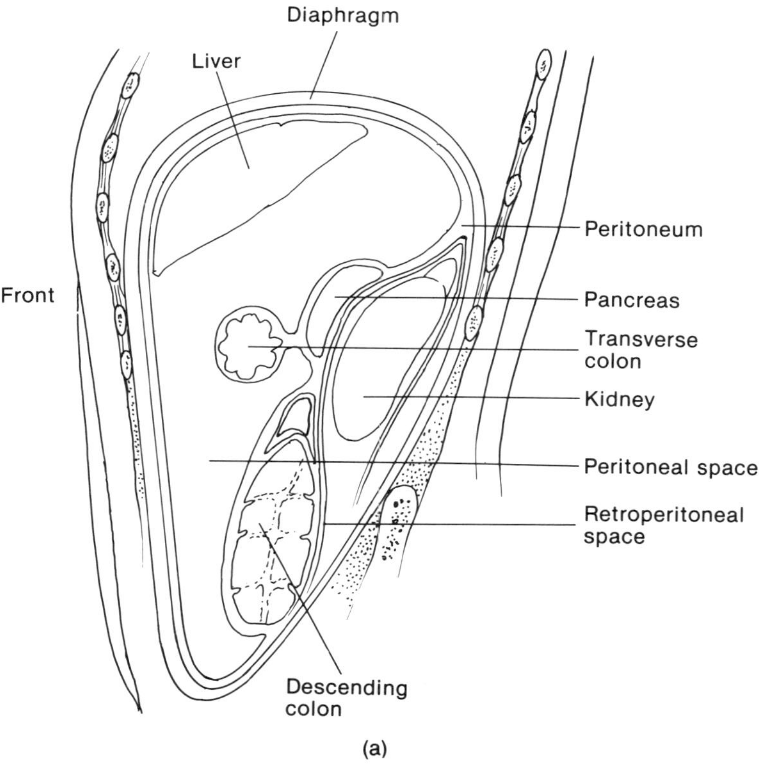

FIGURE 8.1 Peritoneal and retroperitoneal areas of abdominal cavity: (a) side view; (b) cross section.

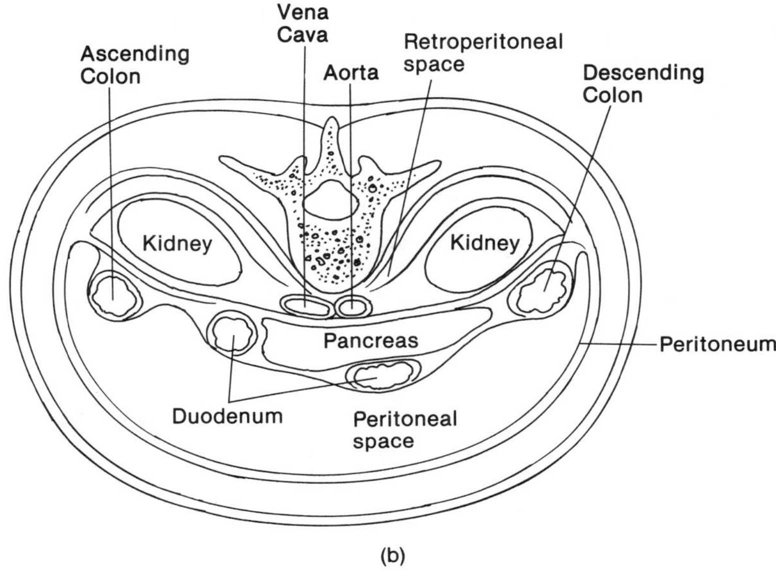

(b)

ANATOMY

The abdomen contains two well-defined anatomic areas: the peritoneal cavity and the retroperitoneal space (Figure 8.1). The peritoneal cavity is lined by a serous membrane called the peritoneum. The layer of peritoneum applied to the muscular walls is known as the parietal peritoneum. The layer that passes over the intra-abdominal organs is called the visceral peritoneum. All organs lined by the peritoneum are said to be intraperitoneal and are contained within the peritoneal cavity. The peritoneum also lines the blood and nerve supply to the intestines, which pass through a structure called the mesentery. The mesentery allows the organs to hang freely in the abdomen.

The pelvic cavity is sometimes regarded as a third space but actually contains both intraperitoneal and retroperitoneal structures.

The diaphragm is a thin, muscular layer that forms a natural division between the abdomen and the chest (Figure 8.2). Remember that the diaphragm moves with breathing, and so the actual division between the chest and abdomen is not constant.

The abdomen may be divided into four quadrants (Figure 8.3). These are often useful in describing areas of pain or signs of trauma.

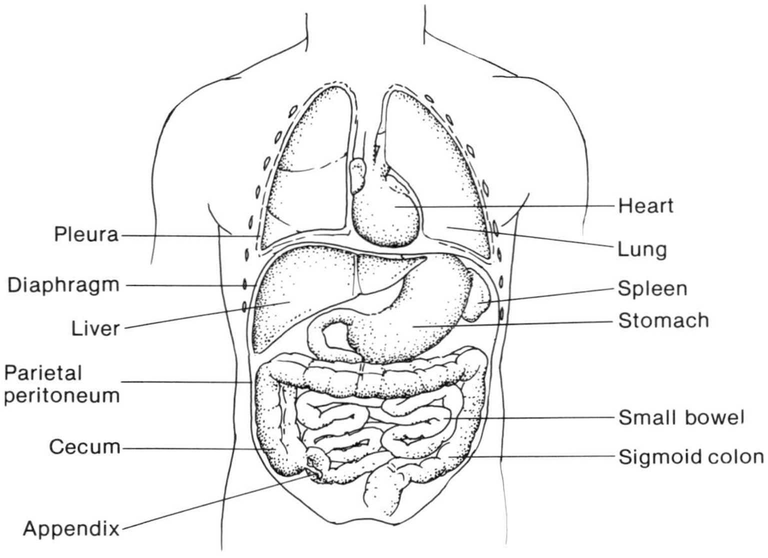

FIGURE 8.2 Note relationship of diaphragm to abdomen and thorax. During full exhalation, diaphragm may rise to the T4–T5 interspace.

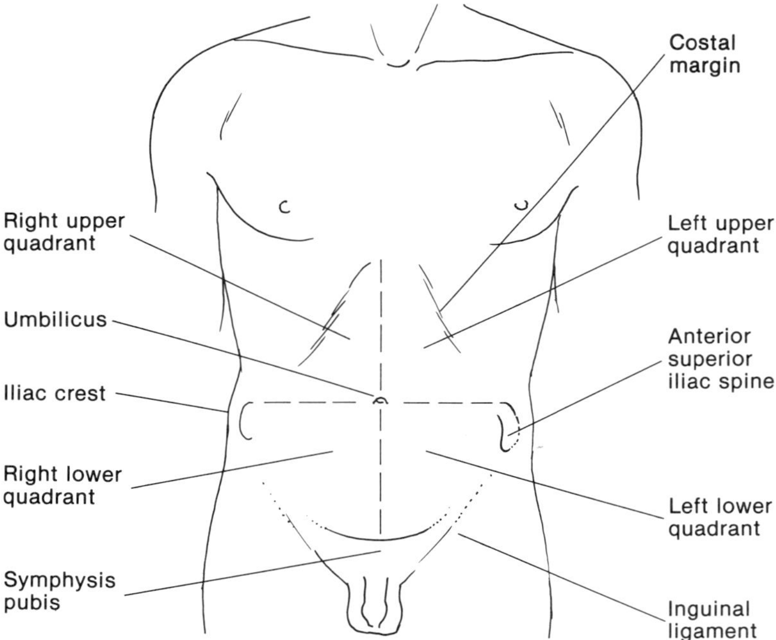

FIGURE 8.3 Abdominal quadrants. This arbitrary configuration aids in describing the location of injuries.

The four quadrants are divided by two perpendicular lines that intersect at the umbilicus. Each quadrant contains noteworthy structures (Table 8.1).

Table 8.1.
Abdominal Organs by Quadrant

Right Upper Quadrant		Left Upper Quadrant	
Liver	(S)	Spleen	(S)
Gallbladder	(H)	Stomach	(H)
Duodenum	(H)	Colon	(H)
Colon	(H)	Pancreas	(S)
Pancreas	(S)	Kidney	(S)
Kidney	(S)		
Right Lower Quadrant		**Left Lower Quadrant**	
Colon	(H)	Colon	(H)
Appendix	(H)	Intestine	(H)
Intestine	(H)	Ureter	(H)
Ureter	(H)	Urinary bladder	(H)
Urinary bladder	(H)		

Key: (H) = hollow
(S) = solid

Hollow Viscera

The organs of the abdominal cavity may be classified as hollow or solid. Hollow organs contain spaces or potential spaces that are usually filled with fluid or a combination of fluid and gas. Hollow organs include the stomach, small intestine, large intestine, rectum, appendix, gallbladder, bile ducts, urinary bladder, and ureters. When injured, hollow organs spill their contents into the peritoneal cavity or retroperitoneal space, causing peritonitis and irritation of the peritoneal lining. In addition, injury to hollow viscera may be accompanied by mesenteric lacerations, which can cause significant bleeding.

The stomach is located in the left and right upper quadrants of the abdomen. Gastric juices are secreted here. Peristalsis of the stomach mixes food and gastric juices together, and protein digestion begins. *Peristalsis* refers to the wave-like contractions of the hollow organs that propel food through the digestive tract. It is these contractions that cause "bowel sounds," noises made by gas and liquids being pushed through a hollow tube. When there is injury to the abdomen, peristalsis may stop and the abdomen becomes silent.

> **Caution!**
> Absent bowel sounds are not a reliable sign of intra-abdominal injury. Don't waste time listening for bowel sounds in the field.

Food passes from the stomach into the small intestines. The latter are divided into three portions: the duodenum, jejunum, and ileum. The approximate length of the small intestine is 20 to 22 feet. The greatest amount of digestion and absorption takes place in the small intestine. All of the small intestine is suspended by mesentery except for the duodenum. The small intestine is connected to the large intestine at the ileocecal valve, or cecum. The large intestine begins at this valve and passes from the right lower quadrant to the right upper quadrant, across to the left upper quadrant and then down to the left lower quadrant, where it takes an S-shaped bend (sigmoid colon) ending in the rectum. The large intestine absorbs water and passes the waste products of digestion through to the rectum where it is stored and then eliminated through the anus. The appendix is a short, tubular structure located in the right lower quadrant. The base of the appendix opens into the cecum. The appendix has no known function in humans.

The gallbladder and bile ducts connect the liver to the duodenum. The gallbladder is just below the liver and functions as a storage place for bile. Bile passes through the bile ducts and enters the small intestine.

The remaining hollow viscera are retroperitoneal. The ureters are hollow tubes that connect the kidneys to the bladder. The ureters act as drains by which urine produced in the kidneys passes downward to the urinary bladder. The urinary bladder is a reservoir for urine prior to its passage from the body through the urethra.

SOLID VISCERA

The solid organs of the abdomen include the liver, spleen, kidneys, pancreas, and adrenal glands. When injured, the solid organs may bleed profusely.

The liver, the largest solid organ in the body, is located beneath the diaphragm in the right upper quadrant of the abdomen. It is somewhat protected by the overlying ribs, but these ribs, if fractured, may in turn lacerate the liver. The liver is vital to life and has many functions, including the production of proteins, clotting factors, and bile; the detoxification of certain substances, including alcohol; and the storage of glycogen.

The spleen is in the left upper quadrant, below the diaphragm and beside and behind the stomach. It is a delicate organ made up of lymphatic tissue, which is very friable and vascular. The spleen filters blood and enhances immunologic resistance to infection.

The pancreas is located in the mid-abdomen with its head in the curve of the duodenum and its tail in the hilum of the spleen. It is a vascular structure that secretes digestive enzymes and bicarbonate into the duodenum. It also contains cells that produce insulin and glucagon. Because of its protected position behind the stomach and over the vertebral column, injuries to the pancreas are unusual. But when they occur, they are very serious.

The kidneys are located retroperitoneally on either side of the spinal column. They produce urine, thereby helping rid the body of waste products, and help to maintain water balance and acid base balance in the body. The kidneys are surrounded by a generous layer of fat that cushions them from injury. The adrenal glands are located above each kidney. These glands produce steroid hormones, which are essential to life.

ASSESSMENT

As an EMT, you must be able to assess the abdomen, identify signs and symptoms, report significant findings, and implement supportive measures as directed by Medical Control. You must also realize that abdominal trauma cannot be managed in the field, because most abdominal problems necessitate definitive care beyond the capability of the EMT. Abdominal injuries, blunt or penetrating, frequently require surgical intervention, and definitive surgical care may be necessary to save the patient's life. With this in mind, let us examine how an EMT provides emergency care to a patient with abdominal trauma.

Caution!
Solid organ injury—think hemorrhage and pain. Hollow organ injury—think contamination and severe pain.

Emergency care is preceded by thorough assessment. This assessment should start as soon as the EMT receives the dispatch information. Mechanism of injury is very important and should be considered early. Scene assessment is also very important. If the patient was involved in a motor vehicle crash, note the type and number of vehicles, the estimated speed, whether restraints were utilized properly, and whether the patient was ejected or required extrication. If the safety belt was worn too loosely, "submarining" may result, with injuries likely to the intestine and lumbar spine. Make note of probable interior vehicle contact points. Falls also cause abdominal trauma, and it is important to know the object from which the fall occurred, its estimated height, the place of landing, the position of the patient when found, the estimated height, and, if available, the cause of the fall. Gunshot wounds and stabbings cause penetrating abdominal trauma. If possible, determine the caliber of the weapon, the number of times it was fired, and at what range. In stab injuries, the size and length of the knife and the position of the assailant would be important in determining the depth and course of wounds. Remember that the majority of abdominal injuries require definitive care, and always be sensitive to the time spent assessing and gathering information.

Begin your physical assessment of the patient with the ABCs —airway, adequacy of breathing, and circulation. After completing the primary survey, begin your secondary assessment with a head-to-toe examination. Verbal, visual, tactile, and acoustical methods of examination are employed simultaneously. Level of consciousness and vital signs are established to form a baseline for future comparison. Using the methods previously described, the examination is completed. Following completion of the physical examination, correlate findings and report the information to Medical Control. Reporting should be conducted in the standard format by objective descriptions. Timely and accurate reporting of information from the patient to the EMT and from the EMT to the physician at Medical Control allows the patient to receive supportive care prior to arrival at the hospital.

Caution!
Assessment of the patient with suspected abdominal injury begins with the ABCs—airway, breathing, and circulation.

MANAGEMENT

Patients with abdominal injury require supportive care. The EMT does not have the means to correct the underlying problem at the scene. If the patient is bleeding internally, stabilization may not be possible and rapid transport becomes the most important consideration. Be highly suspicious of any victim of multi-system trauma. Blood loss into the abdomen or pelvis may be masked by more obvious injuries, only to be manifested later in profound shock or cardiac arrest. Be prepared to care for the patient's immediate needs (airway, ventilation) while being alert to the possibility of subsequent demands.

Caution!
All trauma patients should be considered to have a full stomach. Abdominal trauma may lead to vomiting and aspiration. Be prepared.

Penetrating Injuries

Penetrating injuries to the abdomen usually occur as the result of hostile acts, although self-inflicted wounds are also seen. Penetrating wounds are generally incurred either as stab wounds or bullet wounds. The extent of the damage is difficult to determine at the scene. Penetrating injuries that produce an entrance and exit wound have a high potential for injuring structures that lie in the path of the missile. However, bullets often do not travel in a straight line. The general treatment for penetrating injuries is resuscitation and transport. The provision of oxygen, the establishment of large-bore intravenous lines, and the use of external counterpressure (PASG) may all be appropriate in initial treatment. Be especially careful in using the PASG with a patient at risk for diaphragmatic injury. Inflation of the abdominal compartment may force abdominal organs into the chest cavity, causing further injury and compromising ventilation.

Impaled objects found protruding from the abdomen should not be removed. These objects can create as much (or more) damage on the way out as they did on the way in. Make every effort to stabilize these objects in the position you find them. Secure the object with a bulky dressing, and transport carefully.

Injury of the abdomen may range from minor scratches to lacerations through the abdominal wall leading to evisceration and/or injury to intra-abdominal structures. The omentum and underlying small intestine are the most common structures eviscerated. A moist nonadherent sterile dressing should be placed over the wound and the organs allowed to remain as found.

Blunt Trauma

Care of the patient with blunt trauma depends on the clinical presentation. Again assess the ABCs, complete a secondary survey, and implement supportive measures. Remember, patients may need rapid surgical intervention. Oxygen, intravenous fluids, and external counterpressure may be of value provided contraindication and cautions are kept in mind.

CONCLUSION

Your role in managing patients with abdominal trauma is twofold: First, determine through mechanism of injury and/or clinical assessment which patients are at risk. Second, understand that there is little you can do in the field for these individuals. A high index of suspicion and rapid transport improve outcome.

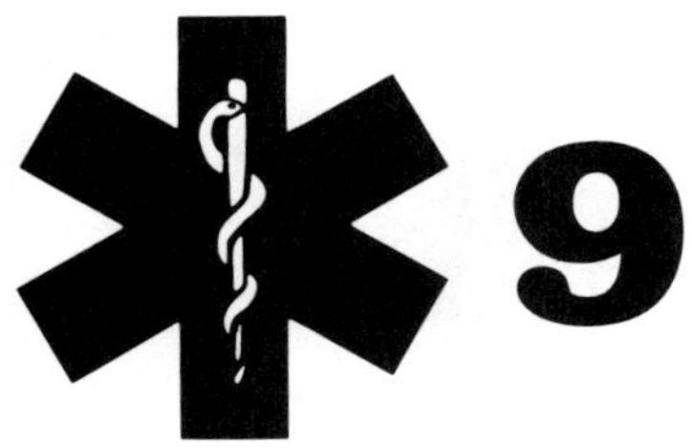

Extremity and Pelvic Fractures

INTRODUCTION

Often, the first injury you will view at the scene is an extremity fracture. The injury is generally easy to spot due to the unnatural alignment of the limb. These injuries can be disabling but are rarely life-threatening. Priorities never change: The ABCs and cervical spine control all come before splinting of fractures. Except for major femur or pelvic fractures, hemorrhagic shock is rarely caused by musculoskeletal trauma. However, in the patient with multisystem trauma, the added bleeding from an injured extremity may tip the balance towards shock.

OBJECTIVES

At the conclusion of this chapter, you should be able to:

1. Recognize the role musculoskeletal injuries play in the patient with multisystem trauma.
2. Summarize extremity fractures in the conscious and unconscious patient based on physical findings.
3. Define the types of fractures and their risks to the patient.
4. Describe dislocation and explain why early management of dislocations is important.

5. Explain hemorrhage control in the care of extremity fractures and the circumstances when a tourniquet is indicated.
6. Describe the management principles for impalement injuries.
7. Explain the principles of fracture splinting, the types of splints, and when they should be used.
8. Describe the proper management of open fractures.
9. Recognize the signs and symptoms of pelvic fractures and their clinical significance.
10. Describe the anatomy of the pelvis and what structures are at risk from pelvic fractures.
11. Explain the mechanism of injury in pelvic fractures, which fractures are most dangerous, and how they are assessed.
12. Explain the principles of PASG use in patients with pelvic fractures.

MUSCULOSKELETAL INJURIES

Fractures

Fracture results when a bone is broken either partially or completely. The fracture may be open or closed. If a fracture is open, the bone end protrudes through the skin or leaves an open wound that communicates with the fracture site. Any patient with a skin laceration close to a fracture site should be considered to have an open fracture. A closed fracture occurs when the bone is broken but the surrounding skin remains intact. Open and closed fractures can cause significant hemorrhage into the soft tissue surrounding the bone. Because an open fracture is contaminated, infection is more likely.

Fractures may also be classified by their configuration (Figure 9.1). A transverse fracture without displacement is less serious than a comminuted fracture with angulation. In the field, the EMT cannot readily distinguish fracture configuration. The most important concern is to recognize the presence of a fracture and prevent further injury.

Dislocation

A dislocation is a condition where the bone comes to lie outside

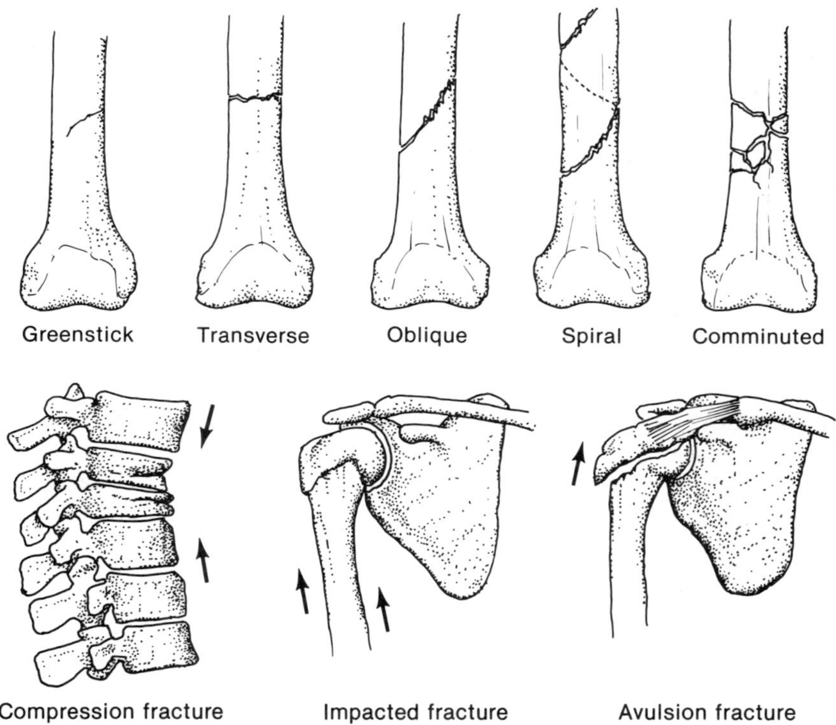

FIGURE 9.1 Fracture type based on configuration of fracture lines.

the joint that normally contains it. A dislocation is usually easy to identify due to the distortion created by the malposition of fragments. Although not immediately life-threatening, joint injuries are emergencies because nerves and blood vessels are often compromised by dislocations. In some instances. early management can prevent amputation. Dislocations are often associated with fractures, causing a fracture-dislocation. Note sensation, color, and pulses distal to the injury. If circulation is compromised, field reduction of the dislocation may be indicated. Medical Control should be sought in this circumstance. Posterior dislocation of the knee is an example of a dislocation suitable for field reduction. Always recheck sensation, color, and pulses after reduction and splinting.

Wounds and Amputations

Open wounds of the extremities can cause massive bleeding, especially following a major arterial laceration. Most bleeding can be controlled by direct pressure, elevation of the extremity, or the use of pressure points. Wounds that have gross contamination, for example, by leaves, gravel, or other debris, should be quickly cleansed and then covered with a sterile dressing.

Amputation is one of the few indications for the use of a tourniquet to control hemorrhage. This injury is disfiguring and may be life-threatening. Pressure should be applied to the stump using a damp sterile dressing and conforming gauze bandage (Kerlex or Kling) or a tightly applied elastic wrap. If the bleeding cannot be controlled in this manner, a tourniquet should be used. Amputated parts should be taken by the EMT to the hospital. Even when the amputated part appears beyond repair, it should be taken to the hospital because a graft may be fashioned from the part. Ideally, the part should be placed in a sterile plastic bag within a plastic bag and then placed on an ice-and-water mix (Figure 9.2). Dry ice should not be used.

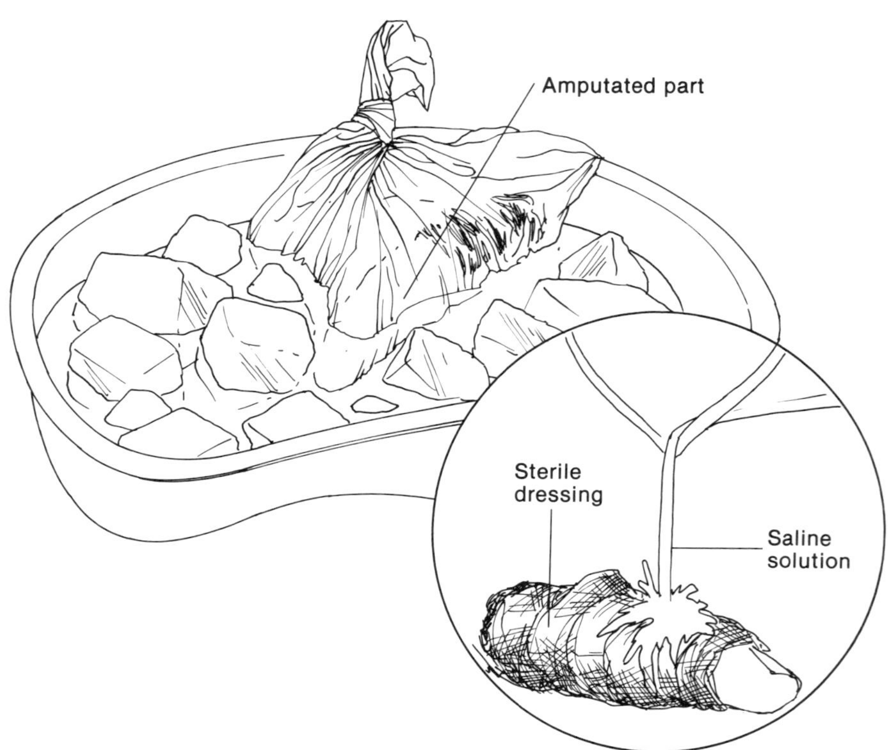

FIGURE 9.2 Proper method of transporting amputated parts.

Impaled Objects

Impaled objects present unique problems to field personnel. It is a time-honored principle that an impaled object should not be removed in the field (Figure 9.3). A bulky dressing should be placed about the object and patients should be transported with the impaled object in place. The operating room is often the safest location for removal of impaled objects, for uncontrolled bleeding may follow. Motion of the impaled object during transport may harm the patient. Immobilization of both patient and impaled object is necessary.

Sprains

A sprain is a partial tear in a ligament supporting a joint. A severe sprain is a nearly complete tear. A complete tear is defined as a torn ligament. In the field, you may be unable to differentiate sprains or ligamentous tears from fractures. Therefore, consider any injury about a joint as a possible fracture.

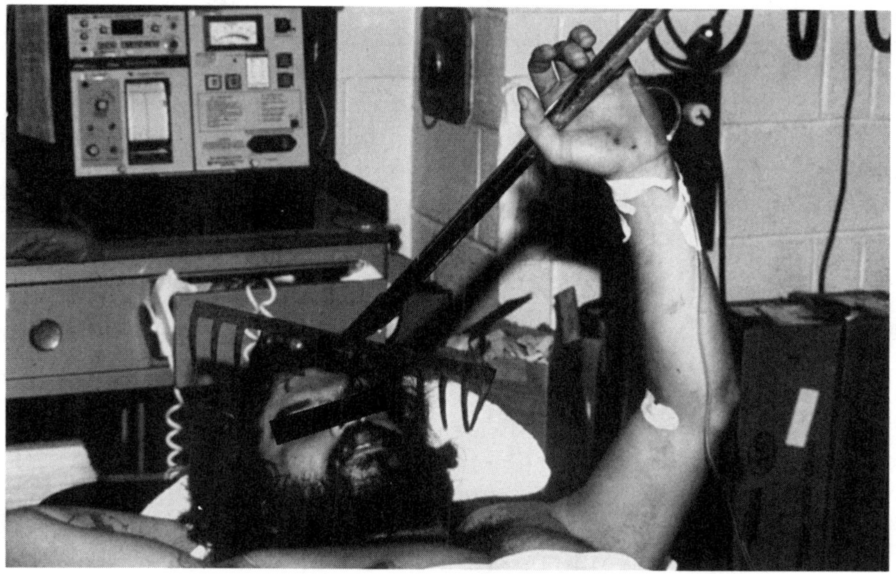

FIGURE 9.3 Garden rake imbedded in skull and frontal lobe of brain. Patient was conscious and held rake handle still during transport!

ASSESSMENT

Once airway, breathing, and circulation have been addressed, a secondary survey should include examination of the extremities and the pelvis. Certain injury patterns are predictable based on associated injuries. For example, a fall in which the patient lands on the feet is associated with lower back injuries. Injuries of the knee should alert you to thoroughly examine the proximal hip. Injuries at the wrist have a higher likelihood of an associated injury at the elbow. This relationship is also true for the ankle and knee. Joints should be evaluated for pain with motion. Distal pulses and sensations should be checked and noted before and after splinting. Crepitus is a very reliable sign of fracture, but it is painful to elicit. Once the suspicion is raised, the extremity should be protected from further motion.

SPLINTING

Splinting is important to decrease pain, and prevent further injury. The objective is to prevent or minimize movement of broken bone ends. Left unsplinted, bone ends will irritate adjacent structures, putting nerves and arteries at risk of further injury. In addition, unsplinted fractures are extraordinarily painful.

In the critically injured patient requiring rapid transport, splinting of the spine alone may be indicated. If the multiple trauma patient has severe injuries to the torso, rapid transport is indicated and additional splinting can be done in the ambulance.

Techniques

Before splinting, cut off clothes rather than pulling them off. Check and record distal pulses and sensation before and after splinting. Check movement distal to the fracture site and mark the pulse with a pen to identify for later confirmation. Only gentle traction should be applied to an angulated fracture to straighten the limb and accommodate splinting. If resistance is encountered, the fracture should be splinted as is.

Open wounds should be covered with a sterile dressing before splints are applied. Do not push bone ends back under the skin in patients with open fractures.

Types of Splints

Splints may be constructed of cardboard, plastic, wood, metal, or other materials. They should be well padded and should extend one joint above and one joint below the injury. Air splints are quite good for lower arm and lower leg fractures. They are also useful for compressing or slowing hemorrhage from an extremity. But remember, it is impossible to monitor pulses through an air splint.

Soft splints such as pillows are good for ankle or foot injuries. A sling and a swathe can be used for a variety of injuries about the upper extremity, including fractures of the clavicle, scapula, upper arm, or elbow. Traction splints are useful to hold alignment of femur fractures, and many types are available. All should be padded with extra material and carefully monitored at the ankle to prevent circulatory insult.

PELVIC FRACTURES

Pelvic fracture is one of the most serious of all injuries to the musculoskeletal system. Patients may rapidly bleed to death at the scene; survivors may be left with considerable long-term disability and alteration of function. Effective field management may save lives and prevent lasting impairment.

ANATOMY OF THE PELVIS

The bony pelvis comprises three bones: the sacrum, the left innominate, and the right innominate. They make up a ring, or more accurately a bucket or tub. Each of the bones is attached to the two bones adjacent to it by very strong ligaments. In the back, the innominate bones are bound to the sacrum by the sacroiliac ligaments. In the front, the two innominate bones are bound together by the pubic symphysis (Figure 9.4). Each of the innominate bones has three parts—the pubis in front, the ileum above and behind, and the ischium below. All converge at the acetabulum, or hip joint socket. In childhood the three bones are separate, but in adulthood they fuse into one large bony half ring. Each of these bones is considered a flat bone; each has a relatively thin cortex and a thick cancellous center. Weight is transmitted down the spine to the sacrum, through the sacroiliac joint to

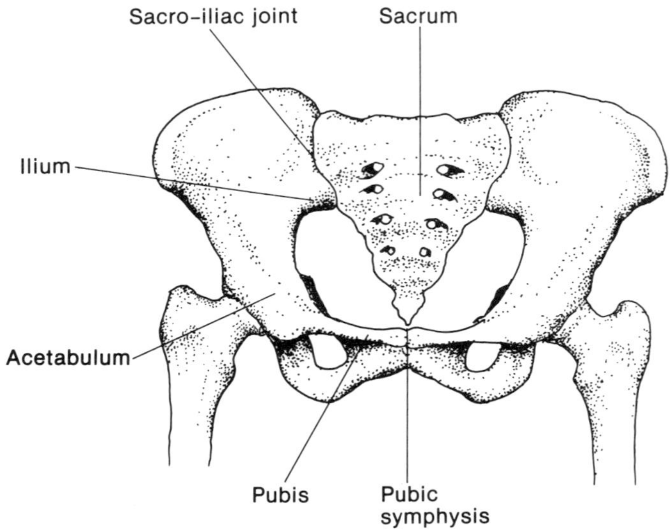

FIGURE 9.4 Anatomy of the pelvic ring.

the strong central bar of the ileum, and down it to the acetabulum. It is then passed across the hip joint into the femur. The anterior portion of the ring helps tie the pelvis together and provides muscle attachment points. The pelvis as a unit is a strong, complex skeletal structure. It is very well suited to its purpose, but it can be severely injured.

The pelvis is very well supplied with blood (Figure 9.5). Through the pelvis pass large vessels to the pelvic enteric organs, the genito-urinary organs, and the lower extremities. These vessels are easily torn when the pelvis is fractured and may bleed severely. The large muscles that control the hip are also well supplied with blood, and injury to the pelvis may result in tearing or lacerating the vessels. The greatest immediate danger from pelvic fractures is severe bleeding and hypovolemic shock. If care is delayed or inadequate, these injuries may result in irreversible shock and death.

Caution!
Pelvic-fracture bleeding may lead to rapid exsanguination without any external evidence of blood loss. If suspected, transport as soon as possible.

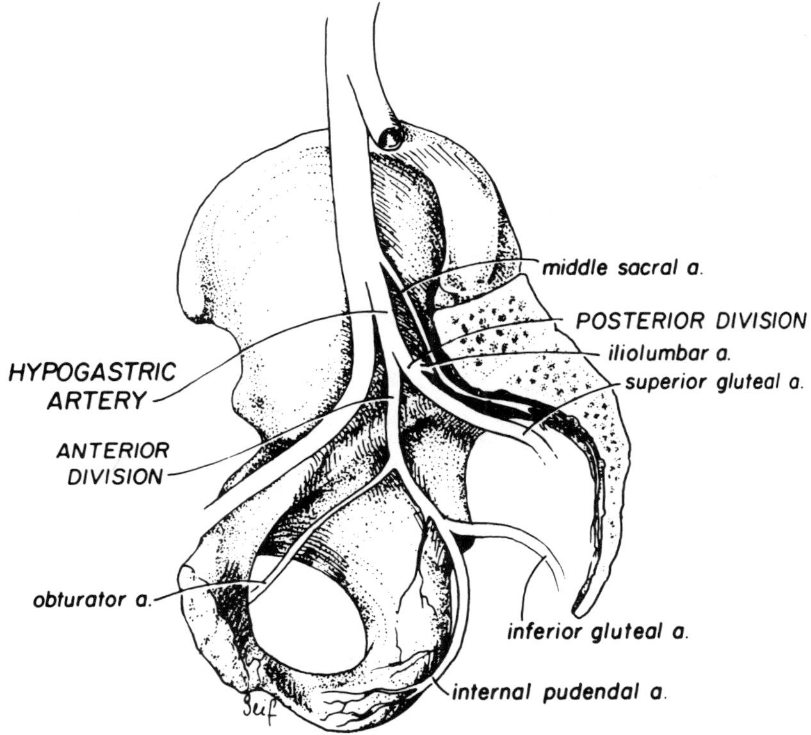

FIGURE 9.5 Blood supply to pelvis.

The pelvis also contains important nerves. Traveling through the sacral portion of the pelvis are the sacral nerve roots, which innervate the pelvic organs and the perineum. The lumbosacral plexus, derived from lumbar roots and sacral roots, gives off the femoral and sciatic nerves. The femoral nerve passes across the anterior pelvic brim and down the front of the thigh. The sciatic nerve passes out the sciatic notch and down the interior of the thigh. The sacral roots are often injured in sacral fractures. Any of the elements of the lumbosacral plexus may be injured by trauma to the sacroiliac joints or posterior ileum. These may be stretching or shearing injuries. The sciatic nerve is often injured by dislocations or fracture-dislocations of the hip or acetabulum.

Large muscle groups cover the pelvis internally and externally. Injury to these muscles may cause profuse bleeding, especially from low-pressure venous oozing, which can fill the retroperitoneal area with blood.

The pelvis contains the ureters, bladder, and urethra, portions of the small and large intestine, the sigmoid colon, and the rectum. In males the prostate gland and the vas deferens are within the pelvis, and the penis, scrotum, and testes are attached to the perineum in front of the pubis. In females the vagina, uterus, fallopian tubes, and ovaries lie within the pelvis.

Injuries to any of these structures can occur with pelvic fractures. Rupture of the bladder is the most common visceral organ injury associated with pelvic fractures. Vaginal or urethral injury may also occur. Rectal injury results in severe contamination and is exceedingly serious.

MECHANISMS OF INJURY

There are several possible mechanisms of injury in pelvic trauma. The mechanism of injury largely determines the type of fracture and/or other injury that occurs. It is helpful to understand injury mechanisms in order to recognize the fractures that result.

Direct Blow

Direct blows to the pelvis are seen in motor vehicle crashes, falls, or pedestrians struck by autos. In these situations either the pelvis is struck by a moving object, such as an auto bumper, or the moving pelvis strikes a nonmoving object, such as the ground or guardrail. Sometimes both may occur in one crash. The severity of the injury is related to the force imparted to the pelvis by the acceleration and/or deceleration and the point of impact.

Penetrating Trauma. These injuries are a special type of direct blow. Penetrating wounds may follow a stabbing, a shooting or impalement. They may cause severe pelvic disruption along with an open wound. Vascular, neurologic, or visceral injury may coexist.

Indirect Blow

Indirect blows occur when the force applied to the pelvis from acceleration and/or deceleration is transmitted through the femur and hip joint. This is caused most often when the knee strikes the dash and stopped by it and the pelvis is then being stopped indirectly through the action of the femur. This most frequently results in dislocation of the hip, fracture of the acetabulum, or both. The pelvic ring may be disrupted as well.

TYPES OF PELVIC INJURY

Several types of injury may result from direct, indirect, or penetrating blows to the pelvis. These may be grouped into several broad categories based on the relationship of the fractured pieces to each other. Severity of injury is influenced by the force of the blow, the structures that are disrupted, and the bony or ligamentous nature of the injury.

Compression

Compression injuries result in an inward collapsing of the pelvis from disruptions of the ring in two or more locations. Visceral injury, such as bladder rupture, may occur. These injuries result in severe instability and may cause significant hemorrhage (Figure 9.6).

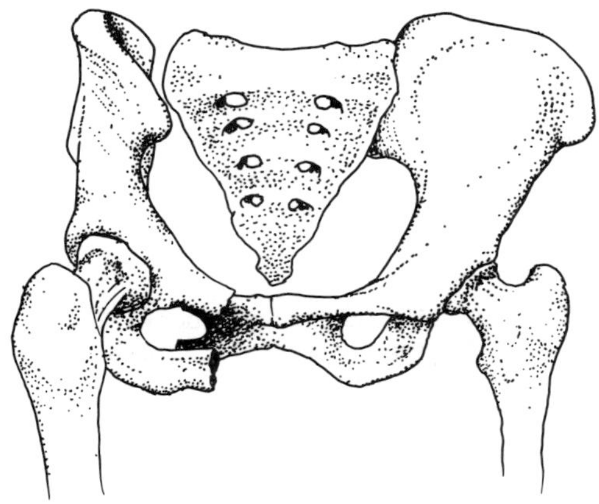

FIGURE 9.6 Lateral compression fracture of the pelvis (unstable).

Shearing

Here, one part of the pelvis is displaced in relationship to the other(s). The displacement may be cephalad–caudad (up and down), anterior–posterior (front to back), or a combination of the two. Bleeding may be massive, and visceral, vascular, and neurologic damage are frequent (Figure 9.7).

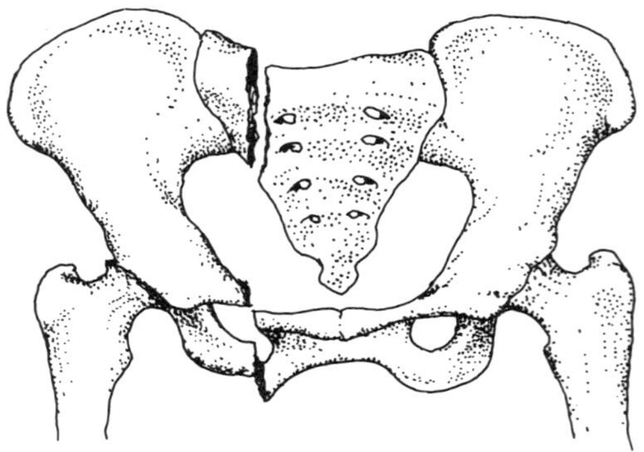

FIGURE 9.7 Vertical shear fracture of the pelvis (unstable).

Open-Book

Open-book injuries are characterized by the pelvis opening up like the two halves of a clam shell. Obviously there must be disruption in at least two points, although one part may be less apparent than the other and act like the hinge. Because the volume of the pelvis is increased, this type of injury may lead to massive bleeding into the opened pelvis (Figure 9.8).

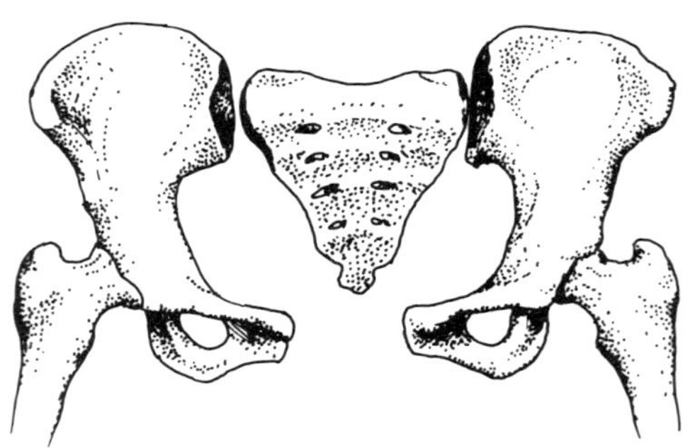

FIGURE 9.8 Open-book fracture—the "spung pelvis" (unstable).

Open Fractures

Although any of the fractures may be associated with a laceration of the skin, the vertical shear fracture associated with deep laceration of the perineum is the most serious. Because the laceration usually communicates with the fracture site, these injuries are especially severe, with mortality approaching 50 percent. The opening to the skin allows blood to escape from the fracture, thus decompressing the tamponaded bleeding and allowing rapid exsanguination. The entry of feces, urine, dirt, and debris causes life-threatening infection and/or long-term disability. These constitute one of the most serious skeletal injuries.

ASSESSMENT

Although a pelvic fracture is not usually as apparent as an amputation, a femoral fracture, or a penetrating chest wound, it can be as serious. Pelvic fractures can usually be assessed (or at least strongly suspected) in the field, and their presence should always be sought, documented, and communicated to Medical Control and treating physicians. A major pelvic disruption dictates that the patient be evacuated rapidly to a trauma center due to the life-threatening nature of the injury and its association with other potentially lethal injuries. For all these reasons, careful assessment for pelvic fracture or disruption is essential in the early stages of field triage and evaluation. A discussion of some of the diagnostic findings in pelvic fractures will help in patient evaluation.

Shock. Since pelvic fractures are very often associated with hypovolemic shock, a pelvic disruption should always be suspected when shock is present. In a major pelvic disruption, a large volume of blood can quickly be lost into the retroperitoneal space, the abdominal cavity, or to the outside. Just as you should think of hemothorax and hemoperitoneum, you should think of pelvic fracture when faced with shock.

Pain. In the conscious or semiconscious patient, the complaint of pain in the pelvis or the ability to elicit pain by pelvic motion indicates a likely pelvic disruption. Treat the painful pelvis as if it were fractured.

Instability. Instability of the disrupted pelvic ring can usually be detected by careful, gentle manipulation of one iliac wing in relation to the other iliac wing (see Chapter 2). The movement may be subtle but is almost always detectable on examination. Avoid this manipulation if the alert patient is already complaining of pelvic pain.

Position and Length of Lower Extremities. Any asymmetry of position or length of the lower extremities should be considered as evidence of a possible pelvic disruption, since excessive external rotation of the thigh, shortening of the lower limb, or adduction, flexion, or even hyperextension of the hip can result.

Open Wounds. The presence of open wounds around the pelvis or in the perineal region should alert you to the possibility of an open pelvic fracture. Sometimes the bone may be exposed, but often it is not.

> **Caution!**
> To determine what is wrong, you must first *think* of the possibilities. Consider the possibility of a pelvic fracture in any patient injured by a high-velocity impact.

Shock, pain, instability, deformity, and open pelvic wounds—when these are identified on the secondary survey, they should call your attention to a possible pelvic fracture.

MANAGEMENT

If you suspect a pelvic fracture, manage the patient as if that were the case. It is far better to overtreat a possible pelvic injury than to fail to stabilize one that is already present. The three most important things in treating a pelvic fracture are (1) *stabilize,* (2) *stabilize,* and (3) *stabilize.* Stay organized.

Check the ABCs first. This unfailing rule should accompany the primary survey and be totally automatic. Then move on to more specific management. Remember that serious pelvic fractures are frequently associated with massive hemorrhage. As much as 20 or 30 units of blood may be lost into the retroperitoneum, the abdomen, or the outside. Therefore, early fluid resuscitation is important. If fluid resuscitation is impossible, the PASG is an excellent way to manage the injured pelvis in the field. PASG application has several simultaneous benefits. The fractured pelvis is stabilized the same way an air splint stabilizes an arm or leg. This decreases movement of the fractured pelvis and diminishes pain and further bleeding. It also helps reduce further soft tissue damage. Second, the PASG can raise systolic pressure by increasing peripheral vascular resistance and myocardial afterload. Third, the PASG helps reduce the volume of the spread pelvis by pushing the two halves back together. This helps tamponade further bleeding into the pelvis and retroperitoneum. The PASG helps with resuscitation, stabilization, and transportation of the patient with pelvic trauma. It should be applied and inflated early in the course of management and maintained until a definitive treatment facility is able to stabilize the patient sufficiently for safe garment removal. The use of PASG is a controversial issue; local medical protocol should be followed.

Caution!
Patients with unstable pelvic fractures should be treated with the same careful immobilization as patients with cervical spine fractures.

Bandage Open Wounds

Any open wounds should be dressed with sterile nonadherent dressings soaked with sterile saline. This is particularly important with exposed viscera. Direct pressure should be applied to areas of active external hemorrhage.

Use a Spine Board

The use of a long spine board with the PASG will give excellent immobilization of the pelvic fracture and is also excellent for immobilizing a fractured femur, knee, or tibia as well. The use of a Thomas, Hare, or Sager splint for a major pelvic disruption offers little or no benefit and may actually further traumatize the pelvis and perineum if you apply it too aggressively.

Evacuate Rapidly

Patients with pelvic disruption need to be evacuated as soon as practical to a facility capable of treating victims of serious trauma. It is often these patients for whom the first hour is truly "golden"; delay in treatment may adversely affect their outcome.

CONCLUSION

Patients with multi-system trauma and extremity fractures present a challenge. Resist being drawn to the most obvious injury, usually the painful and deformed arm or leg. Proper care of extremity injuries is important to relieve pain and prevent further injury. Remember to stay organized and address the ABCs first. Although extremity injuries may appear severe, they are not usually life-threatening. The surgical axiom "For the want of a limb, a life should not be lost" applies to field care of multi-trauma victims.

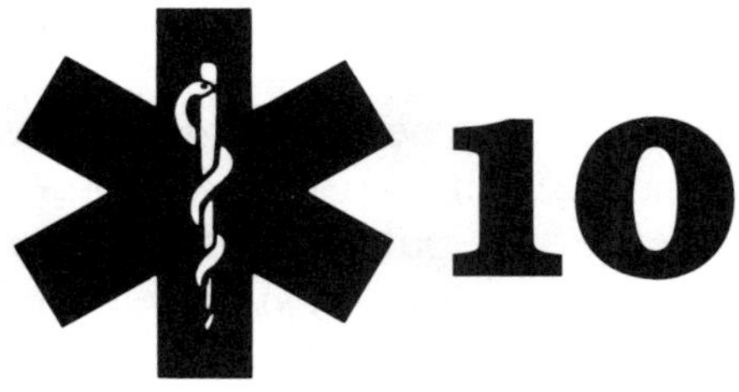

Trauma in Pregnancy

INTRODUCTION

Trauma is the leading cause of death in women during most of their reproductive years and accounts for more than twice as many deaths in women as the total maternal mortality. During pregnancy, most women remain active and ambulatory, and are thereby vulnerable to both major and minor injuries. Trauma of some type affects approximately 6 to 7 percent of expectant mothers and peaks during the third trimester.

The approach to the pregnant and nonpregnant patient is basically identical. But a number of anatomic and physiologic changes during pregnancy call for special consideration in the prehospital setting.

OBJECTIVES

At the end of this chapter, you should be able to:

1. Demonstrate knowledge of the anatomic and physiologic changes of pregnancy.
2. Understand the implication of both blunt and penetrating abdominal trauma and their risks to mother and baby.
3. Demonstrate simple methods to improve the cardiopulmonary status of the mother in the field.

An injury to a pregnant woman is a stressful event for the EMT. Not only is there the usual concern about the injured patient, but there is an additional awareness that the baby is at risk, *and* this awareness is greatest in the victim. This often translates into errant judgment by the mother, who wants to do everything possible for the baby without recognizing that compromising her own status is what will most jeopardize the baby.

> **Caution!**
> The leading cause of fetal mortality is maternal mortality. By doing what is best for the mother, you improve the baby's outcome.

Trauma to an expectant mother calls for firmness and reassurance. Few other field situations will tax your professionalism as much.

Women can be pregnant and not know it. Women can also know they are pregnant and deny it. Therefore, injury to a young woman should always be viewed in the context of her possibly being pregnant. If the patient is conscious and oriented, ask simple questions: "Are you pregnant?" or "Is there a possibility of your being pregnant?" If the patient is not following commands, don't overlook the possibility that she may be pregnant. Resuscitation priorities are the same, but certain anatomic and physiologic changes will affect how the pregnant patient responds to the stress of trauma.

ANATOMY OF PREGNANCY

Early pregnancy offers little external clue to the casual observer. At 12 weeks' gestation, the uterus still remains confined to the pelvis but may be palpated at the pubis (Figure 10.1). The fundus of the uterus reaches the umbilicus by 20 weeks and the costal margin by 36 weeks. Thereafter, the baby descends into the pelvis, and the abdominal configuration may actually appear less protuberant at term (40 weeks). Both the risk of fetal injury and the survivability of fetal injury increase with gestational age. Early in pregnancy, the fetus is surrounded by amniotic fluid, cushioned by a thick uterine wall, and protected by the bony confines of the pelvis. By the third trimester, the relative volume of fetus to am-

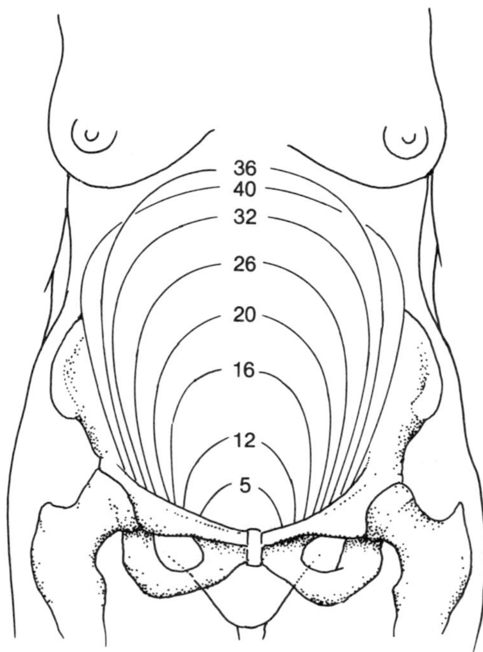

FIGURE 10.1 Uterine size by week of gestation.

niotic fluid has changed, the uterine wall has thinned considerably, and most of the body of the fetus lies exposed above the pelvis. Despite this less favorable environment, maturity of the fetus is even more important in the ability of the baby to survive following an injury to itself or to the uterus.

As the uterus enlarges, it encroaches upon other structures related to it. The usual contents of the abdomen are pushed upward, compressing the stomach and intestines. Gastric emptying is delayed and vomiting is more likely.

The uterus also compresses the ureters and adjacent vascular structures, of which the inferior vena cava (IVC) is by far the most clinically pertinent. IVC compression is directly correlated to field care of the patient. If the patient is in the supine position, IVC compression can reduce the volume of blood returning to the heart. In a hypovolemic patient, this can be a critical factor in reducing cardiac output and further compromising perfusion. IVC compression can also increase venous pressure in the pelvis, including pressure in the placental circulation. If traumatic disruption of the placenta has taken place, increased placental congestion can result in loss of the baby.

All pregnant patients with an enlarged uterus palpated at or above the umbilicus should be transported on the left side, *provided* spinal injury is not suspected. If the patient must be transported supine, the EMT should gently manually displace the uterus to the left side and elevate the right hip. This position should be monitored throughout transport.

> **Caution!**
> Relieving uterine pressure on the inferior vena cava is a simple but vital maneuver in the injured pregnant patient.

PHYSIOLOGY OF PREGNANCY

The maternal changes of pregnancy are designed to provide an optimal environment for the fetus to develop. In part, this environment occurs anatomically. The physiologic alterations increase the mother's ability to provide this optimal environment. The EMT needs to understand these changes and recognize that what is abnormal in the nonpregnant state may be normal during pregnancy, and vice versa.

Vital Signs

Heart Rate. Pulse rate increases throughout pregnancy, reaching a rate of 15 to 20 beats per minute faster than the resting state during the third trimester.

Blood Pressure. Blood pressure, both systolic and diastolic, falls during the second trimester by 5 to 15 mmHg. By the time of delivery, blood pressure returns nearly to normal.

Cardiovascular Performance. Alterations in vital signs are associated with underlying changes in blood volume and cardiac output. Blood volume increases throughout pregnancy. At 34 weeks' gestation, blood volume may reach 50 percent above what is normal in the prepregnant state. This increase is largely in plasma volume, resulting in the artificially low hemoglobin and "anemia" of pregnancy. Cardiac output increases more rapidly and may be 1 to 1.5 liters a minute above normal before uterine enlargement is apparent clinically.

These changes are important. Because the pregnant patient has an expanded volume, she can tolerate a greater acute loss of blood than her nonpregnant counterpart. Yet, the vascular bed that is most sensitive to epinephrine and norepinephrine release is the placenta. So, even if the mother is bleeding but giving the appearance of tolerating her injury, the fetus may be profoundly compromised. These changes in the mother require careful interpretation. Anticipate problems even though the mother is "stable."

Caution!
The baby may be in trouble before the mother becomes unstable. Manage all injured pregnant patients as if they are about to "crash."

Placenta

The placenta reaches its maximal size at 36 to 38 weeks. It does not contain elastic tissue, so it cannot contract. Placental circulation is maximally dilated throughout pregnancy. Direct trauma to the placenta leads to bleeding, compromised blood supply to the fetus, and the release of tissue thromboplastin and other factors that produce thrombosis.

Placental separation is the leading cause of fetal loss if the mother survives. Tearing or separation of the placenta follows shearing forces to the uterus that cause a maldistribution of forces between the elastic and vascular uterus and the inelastic placenta. Direct trauma to the uterus is not necessary to cause placental separation, which may instead follow isolated deceleration.

MATERNAL INJURIES

Pelvic fracture is the most common injury to the mother that causes loss of the baby. It may involve the three mechanisms of maternal shock, placental separation, and direct fetal injury. Fracture of the fetal skull with intracranial hematoma is the most common cause of death.

Blunt injury to the mother and fetus can be reduced by properly worn three-point restraints. The three-point restraint prevents the harmful jackknifing seen with the lap belt alone.

Penetrating trauma may be seen in pregnant women. Fetal survival following penetrating trauma is related to fetal maturity and site of injury. An abdominal wound outside the uterus will likely cause extensive vascular and/or intestinal injury, since the enlarging uterus compresses surrounding organs. Sixty percent of the bullets that strike the uterus will would the fetus. This causes high fetal mortality but low maternal mortality.

MANAGEMENT

As is true for all injured patients, prevent further injury to the mother *and* to the baby. Even though the mother may not appear badly injured, anticipate that the baby is in difficulty. Fetal distress is difficult to assess even in a relatively controlled environment. The field is not the place to search for subtle findings or changes in heart tones. Assume that the situation is urgent and transport the patient immediately. Supply oxygen, transport the patient on her left side or with her right hip elevated and the uterus manually displaced to the left side.

Transmit pertinent clinical data over the radio. An obstetrician is needed in virtually all instances of trauma during pregnancy, and this need may be more promptly addressed if the situation is known ahead of time. Sophisticated fetal monitoring equipment may be made available with advance notice to the emergency department.

CONCLUSION

Do no further harm to the patient(s). Recognize that the fetus will be affected before the mother shows signs of shock. Anticipate instability—transport the patient on her left side, or manually displace the uterus to the left. Provide oxygen, and notify the hospital by radio of the patient's status.

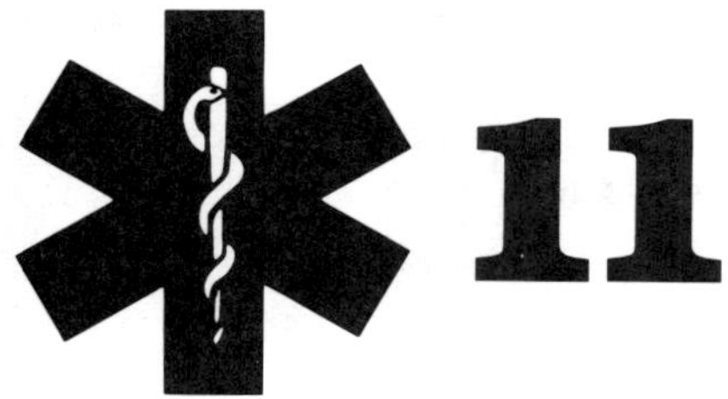

11

Pediatric Trauma

INTRODUCTION

Trauma is the leading cause of death in children. Accidental death is four times more prevalent than any other childhood disease. The leading causes of childhood trauma death are listed in Table 11.1. Blunt trauma accounts for almost 90 percent of injuries in children. Motor vehicle crashes as occupant and pedestrian account for almost half the deaths. The "three-level injury snydrome" affecting the unrestrained driver has a counterpart in child pedestrian impacts. When a child is struck by a car the most common combination of injuries is lower extremity, abdomen, and head. This is due to the bumper striking the thigh, the fender hitting the abdomen, and the child being thrown and striking the head. Head trauma accounts for the highest proportion of blunt injuries in children (Table 11.2), and a higher proportion than in the adult population. Falls are also a common cause of death, and head injury is the major consequence in the fall. Penetrating trauma is less common, but accidental wounding by firearms—an all too common tragedy—often ends fatally. Many such incidents are preventable.

Table 11.1
Leading Causes of Trauma Deaths in Children

• Motor vehicle related	45%
• Drowning	16%
• Burns	16%
• Firearms	3%
• Falls	3%
• Other	18%

Source: National Safety Council, *Accident Facts,* 1989 ed.

Table 11.2
Distribution of Blunt Injuries in Children

Head	63%
Extremities	29%
Abdomen	14%
Chest	9%

OBJECTIVES

At the completion of this chapter, you should be able to:

1. Define differences in response to injury between child and adult.
2. List the common causes of childhood trauma deaths and anatomic areas commonly affected by blunt injury.
3. Distinguish the field approaches to critical and noncritical injuries in children.
4. Discuss chest injuries in children and how they are recognized in the field.
5. Define variations in vital signs and relate them to age of the patient.
6. Summarize the theory of the Pediatric Trauma Score and its usefulness in field management.
7. Explain the important principles of childhood head trauma management.

SPECIAL CONSIDERATIONS IN CHILDHOOD TRAUMA

Panic is the enemy of the prehospital care professional. When approaching an injured child, it is important to control your own emotions. Not only is the patient injured and upset, but parents, family members, and bystanders often must be calmed. You must enter the scene armed with knowledge and confidence in order to minimize the emotional impact of the situation.

Physiologic Considerations

Blood volume is proportionally 20 to 25 percent larger in children than in adults. However, the actual blood volume is much smaller. Although loss of up to 30 percent of blood volume may not cause significant change in vital signs, bloos loss considered modest in the adult may be rapidly fatal in the child. Ranges for vital signs (Table 11.3) vary with age and should be used only as guidelines, not as rules. Perfusion, level of consciousness, number of injuries, and body temperature are other useful determinants.

Table 11.3
Vital Signs by Age in Children

	Blood Pressure (mmHg)	Heart Rate (beats/min)	Respiration Rate (breaths/min)
Infant	80	160	40
Child	90	140	30
Adolescent	100	120	20

Practical Tips

One of the first things you must do is gain the confidence of the parents. A good working knowledge and the proper equipment will help you demonstrate competence and control. Do not try to separate the family. Instead, make the parent or family member an active part of emergency medical care. Delegate simple tasks to them and explain what you are doing for their child.

Use appropriate language for the child's age and make a game out of your assessment. Note changes in consolability as you assess.

If you were originally able to quiet the child or distract the child and can no longer do so, suspect a decreasing level of consciousness, pain, hypoxia, or shock.

There are many tricks in dealing with children. Do not ask the children if they want something done—they won't. Instead, explain what you are going to do, and be honest about pain and when it will be over. Get on your knees and down to their level. Use the parent to help in packaging—for example, by putting on the blood pressure cuff. This may help alleviate the child's concern about pain.

Remember that you must have the parents' permission to manage the child. Keep them on your side. If parents refuse you permission to care for or transport their child, explain to them the need for care and document their refusal. If possible, have them sign a refusal form.

When a parent is not available or also injured, you must manage the patient according to local laws and protocol if an emergency exists. Do not hesitate to transport, and notify Medical Control of the situation.

ASSESSMENT AND MANAGEMENT

The dispatch information may provide important clues to look for as you approach the scene. Look for dangers to the rescuers or to the patient, search for the mechanism of injury, and inspect environmental factors.

Primary Survey

- *A*irway with C-spine control
- *B*reathing
- *C*irculatory status (shock, major bleeding)
- *D*isability (level of consciousness)
- *E*xposure (skin temperature and environment)

Determine whether the child's injuries are critical. If they are, place the child on a backboard with cervical spine immobilization, transport immediately, provide lifesaving interventions and a secondary survey en route, and contact Medical Control. If the situation is not critical, place the patient on a backboard with C-spine immobilization, perform a secondary survey, transport, and contact Medical Control.

Airway and Cervical Spine Immobilization. The jaw thrust maneuver with in-line stabilization is recommended for opening the airway. Always assume that the cervical spine is injured. Do not hyperextend the neck. Remember that the occiput of the child is relatively larger, may cause passive flexion of the neck, and tends to occlude the airway.

Breathing. Look, listen, feel for breathing. Is air moving? If not, initiate rescue breathing. If the child is breathing, evaluate the adequacy of air exchange and look for signs of distress. Can the child speak, cry, or grunt? Check the chest for symmetrical rise and fall. Use a stethoscope to check for bilateral breath sounds. Look at the chest for suprasternal or intercostal retractions. Observe for open wounds or bruises over the chest wall.

When emergency ventilation is necessary, mouth to mask may be attempted. Give low-pressure breaths that barely cause the chest to rise. Breathing rates vary with age (Table 11.3). A self-inflated bag may be suitable for some children. Use a non-pop-off valve-type bag. In near drowning, hypercarbia, or aspiration, high pressure may be required.

Circulation. Capillary refill is the easiest, quickest, and most reproducible way to assess circulation in the child. Compress the nail bed and release to see how quickly the blood returns. Color normally returns to the blanched area in one to two seconds. Any delay suggests impaired circulation.

Blood pressure in most cases must be obtained by palpation using a cuff that snugly fits the patient's arm. Find the radial pulse, pump up the cuff, and note the level at which the pressure returns. Blood pressure and heart rate vary with age (Table 11.3). As a rule of thumb, normal blood pressure should be 80 plus twice the patient's age. Know the normal values so that you can interpret findings in the patient.

Caution!
Regardless of age, trends in vital signs are most important in clinical assessment of the patient.

Shock. Shock in the injured child is hypovolemic until proven otherwise. Hypovolemic shock results from blood loss, which can be caused by internal injuries from fractures or lacerations. Profound shock may occur in a short period from relatively small blood loss. The key to effective shock management is anticipation. Stop external blood loss by direct pressure, elevation, or pressure points. *Use your hands.*

> **Caution!**
> Internal bleeding cannot be controlled in the field. Rapid transport to a suitable hospital is the only effective treatment.

Signs of shock are as follows:

- capillary refill delayed longer than two seconds
- pale, cool, and damp skin
- rapid, weak pulse
- decreased level of consciousness
- rapid, shallow respirations
- blood pressure less than 80 mmHg

Total blood volume is based on weight—40 ml/lb. Early signs and symptoms of shock develop with a 20 percent decrease in blood volume. Falling blood pressure is a late sign of shock.

Treatment of shock. Direct pressure is the quickest and most effective way of stopping external bleeding and preventing shock. Compress a pressure point to slow bleeding, and elevate the extremity. Apply a tourniquet only as a last resort; document the time it is applied, and if possible contact Medical Control.

If blood pressure falls below 80 mmHg systolic, consider inflating the PASG. A pediatric garment should be used when circumstances indicate. For children under 10, the abdominal compartment should not be inflated because of possible compromise of ventilation.

In brief, the initial assessment and management of the injured child should include these measures:

- maintain the airway.
- assume C-spine injury and use inline traction.

- administer high-flow oxygen.
- check capillary refill and blood pressure.
- if necessary, apply PASG and inflate to maintain 80 systolic.
- evaluate neurologic status.
- conserve body heat.
- transport to appropriate hospital.

Secondary Survey

The secondary survey of the injured child is a rapid head-to-toe evaluation for major injury. If an emergent condition warrants rapid transport, the secondary survey can be done en route.

Pediatric Trauma Score (PTS). The PTS (Table 11.4) is a tool for determining injury severity and transport destinations. Children with a PTS of 6 or less require care in hospitals with specialized pediatric trauma capabilities.

Table 11.4
Pediatric Trauma Score

Component	+2	+1	−1
Size	>20 kg	10–20 kg	≤10 kg
Airway	Normal	Maintainable	Unmaintainable
Systolic BP	>90 mmHg	50–90 mmHg	≤50 mmHg
CNS	Awake	Obtunded/LOC	Coma/decerebrate
Open wound	None	Minor	Major/penetrating
Skeletal	None	Closed fracture	Open/complex fracture

Head Injuries. Because of the major role head injury plays in childhood trauma, care of children with head trauma is exceedingly important. The major focus of field head trauma is to prevent secondary brain injury (by aggressively managing hypoxia and hypotension) and prevent cervical spine injury (by careful handling and proper immobilization). Protect the cervical spine as you maintain the airway. Give 100 percent oxygen immediately. It is blood that carries oxygen to the brain, so keep the blood pressure up.

Do a brief neurologic check. Rate the level at which the patient responds:

A—alert

V—responds to verbal stimulus

P—responds only to pain

U—unresponsive

Unless the patient is in shock, a 30° elevation of the head of the spine board may help lower intracranial pressure. Do not compromise the cervical spine when elevating the head. The depth and rate of ventilation should be increased. This will constrict blood vessels and reduce intracranial pressure.

Assess and reassess the level of consciousness. Note and report any change to Medical Control. Pupil assessment should be done and noted in the chart. Note whether the eyes are moving together, moving opposite, or set in one position.

Intracranial bleeding in a small infant can result in enough blood loss to cause shock. This is the one exception to the rule that shock is not caused by intracranial injury. However, in the majority of pediatric cases shock originates elsewhere. Increased intracranial pressure is dangerous and may lead to the following signs and symptoms:

- altered level of consciousness
- weakness on one side of the body
- vomiting
- dilation of one pupil
- hypertension
- slow pulse
- irregular respirations or apnea

Chest Injuries.

Simple pneumothorax. Pneumothorax is usually accompanied by collapse of the lung. It is the most common chest injury in children. The mechanism of injury may be blunt or penetrating. Because of the elasticity of the chest wall in children, rib fractures are far less common than in the adult. Nonetheless, severe chest injury does occur without rib fractures. Symptoms include:

- pain in chest with breathing
- decreased breath sounds on affected side
- external injuries (contusions)
- subcutaneous emphysema

- tachypnea
- dyspnea
- cyanosis
- hypotension
- bradycardia

Tension pneumothorax. A tension pneumothorax may develop if air enters the pleural space from the lung or through the chest wall and cannot escape. The lung collapses, and the same symptoms and signs develop as in simple pneumothroax. However, tension pneumothorax is more serious because it elevates intrathoracic pressure and interferes with filling of the heart. Deviation of the trachea to the side opposite the tension is an additional clue, as is distention of neck veins, but these may not be discernible in the field.

Hemothorax. A hemothorax develops when blood accumulates in the pleural space. Generally, this is due to a tear in a blood vessel in the chest wall or to a lacerated lung. What would be considered an insignificant hemothorax in the adult can cause profound shock in children because of their relatively small blood volume. Hemothorax symptoms are similar to pneumothorax symptoms, but the principal problem is blood loss. Shock is more likely.

Other forms of chests injury (flail chest, pericardial tamponade) occur in children but are uncommon. See Chapter 4—Trauma for a more complete explanation of these injuries.

Management of chest injury. Open chest wounds (open pneumothorax, or sucking wounds of the chest) should be managed in the field. First close the wound using petrolatum gauze or the inner surface of the foil packaging. Observe for subsequent tension, and release the dressing periodically if you suspect it. Maintain the airway, breathing, and circulation. Provide 100 percent oxygen by mask.

Abdominal Injuries. The liver and spleen both protrude below the rib margin in children and thus are vulnerable to blunt injury. Bleeding can intially be brisk. As the blood pressure drops and blood flow to the abdominal organs decreases, so does the rate of blood loss. A clot may form. However, bleeding may resume during movement. A delicate but urgent load-and-go situation exists in children with these injuries. Remember, patients with abdominal injuries tend to vomit.

> **Caution!**
> Patient should be on spine board with C-spine immobilized to allow safe turning in case of vomiting.

Extremity Injuries. Most extremity fractures in children can be splinted as in the adult. Be sure to check the pulse before and after splinting, and note your findings in the record. Reassess the fracture site from time to time for changes in color, skin temperature, and perfusion. If a child is in an infant car seat, it is generally safe to transport him or her as is. Tape the infant securely to the seat before moving it.

Burns. Each year 60,000 children are hospitalized for burns. Many more are injured but do not require hospital care. There is little to do for the burn victim except to transport. However, there are several things not to do. Because the child has a greater surface area per body weight, burns quickly result in heat loss. Do not apply ice or cold dressings during transport; hypothermia can occur quickly. Do not apply ointments or other medication to the burn, for these will require removal at the hospital. Do not delay transport. Volume depletion can occur quickly in children with serious burns. Early resuscitation with fluids is essential to survival.

CONCLUSION

Children are not little adults; they have different anatomic, physiologic, and psychologic reactions to injury. A reassuring approach is essential to reducing anxiety in both child and parent. The ability to reassure will be based on your competence in dealing with injured children.

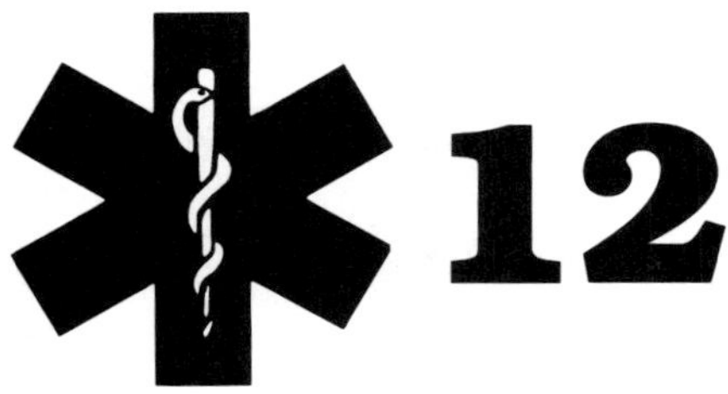

Environmental Hazards

INTRODUCTION

American society is mobile and recreation-oriented. Whether at work or at play, people are subject to a great number of environmental hazards. The list is almost endless. This chapter describes the more important hazards, along with their possible consequences for both victim and rescuer. Certain emergencies that are particularly dangerous to the rescuer are discussed in detail, with the emphasis always on safety for both parties. Although it is impossible to anticipate all emergencies provoked by our environment, you should find the following information and principles useful.

OBJECTIVES

At the conclusion of this chapter, you should be able to:

1. Recognize the signs and symptoms of diving illness.
2. Summarize the basic pathophysiology of diving illness and why specialized care is needed.
3. Recognize the necessity of immediate airway control and rescue breathing in victims of near drowning.
4. Describe why trauma and hypothermia are commonly encountered in patients with near drowning.

5. Describe common poisonous snakes and spiders and how to identify them.
6. Explain basic emergency medical care for snake and spider bites.
7. Recognize the principles of distance and dilution when dealing with hazardous or radioactive materials.
8. Recognize the complex nature of hazardous materials and radioactivity and know where to seek further assistance.
9. Explain the pathophysiology of heat and cold injury.
10. Describe signs and symptoms of heat and cold injury and the way to initiate immediate treatment.
11. Explain how to determine the extent of burn injury and whether airway injury exists.
12. Explain the principles of immediate burn care.

BAROTRAUMA

Each year several million people participate in sport diving. Many of these people fly home within hours of a dive. Thus, although barotrauma—illness caused by breathing compressed air underwater—is more common near the seacoast and in warmer climates, it may appear in an area where sport diving is uncommon. A brief medical history will often provide the information necessary to suspect diving illness.

Barotrauma is caused by the increase in atmospheric pressure as a diver submerges. For each 33 feet of descent, the diver's body is exposed to an increase of one atmosphere of pressure (760 torr). As ambient pressure increases, all body structures are compressed, but the gas in the diver's body is compressed to a much greater extent than the liquid or solid structures. It is this tendency of gases to change volume in relationship to pressure that causes most diving injuries.

The compressed air that divers breathe contains a large percentage of nitrogen. As ambient pressure increases with descent, nitrogen is forced into the blood and the tissues in increasing concentrations. In sufficient concentration, nitrogen is an anesthetic and will cause nitrogen narcosis, or "rapture of the deep." This condition is characterized by drunken behavior—poor judgment, loss of coordination, hallucination, and disorientation. Drowning because of impaired judgment is a major hazard.

The treatment for nitrogen narcosis is to ascend to the surface, where the excess nitrogen can be "blown off" through the lungs. The high concentration of nitrogen that is forced into the blood and tissues as the diver descends will begin to exit the tissues as the diver ascends and the ambient pressure decreases. But if ascent is too rapid, nitrogen will appear in tissue and blood as free bubbles rather than as gas dissolved in liquid. This problem is avoided by ascending slowly.

Types of Decompression Sickness

The "Bends." When bubbles accumulate in blood and tissue, they cause a range of problems known as decompression sickness (DCS). "Bends," the most common malady, represents 60 to 75 percent of all decompression illness. "Bends" is caused by bubble accumulation in the joints and appears as severe joint pain soon after a dive. The affected joints will be painful out of proportion to the physical signs of injury, which are minimal. Palpation of the joints will not dramatically increase the pain. The diver may flex or bend the joints in an attempt to relieve the pain. A rash may mottle the chest, abdomen, forearms, and thighs. Severe pain occurs in the area of the rash, which is slightly tender to palpation. The rash itself is of no long-term importance, but it is a sign of DCS.

The "Chokes." The "chokes," or gas bubbles in lung tissue, may occur as long as 12 hours after a dive; this is the second most common form of DCS. The diver experiences tight substernal chest pain, usually worsened by a deep breath. The pain does not radiate into the arms or jaws. A cough is a prominent symptom. At first it is controllable, but later it becomes uncontrollable and occurs in paroxysms. Dyspnea is a common complaint. The physical examination of the patient is usually normal; the lungs are clear when auscultated, and heart tones are normal.

Spinal Cord DCS. This occurs when nitrogen bubbles appear in the spinal cord. Frequently the patient notices back pain followed by weakness or numbness in some or all extremities. Total paralysis may occur, and fecal or urinary incontinence is not uncommon because neurologic control of sphincter muscles is lost. These patients appear to have had a stroke!

Air Emboli

The gas in the lungs, sinuses, and ears at the bottom of the descent will expand as the diver ascends. Unless the ascent is safe, the expanding gas may rupture the structures that enclose it, causing ear or sinus pain. Most dangerous to the diver is rupture of the lung itself. A pneumothorax or pneumomediastinum may occur, or air may enter the central circulation and be expelled from the heart only to embolize in the peripheral circulation. Most often air emboli cause a strokelike syndrome as they enter the brain circulation, or cardiac arrest from embolization of the coronary arteries. These symptoms occur within 15 to 20 minutes of surfacing.

Assessment and Treatment

All patients with DCS or air embolus symptoms require rapid medical evaluation. The key to assessing these disorders is the history of recent sport diving. If you suspect DCS or air embolus, administer 100 percent oxygen through a face mask and transport the patient to an appropriate hospital immediately. All DCS or air embolus victims will require treatment in a decompression chamber. The Diving Accident Network provides 24-hour-a-day information about diving-related injuries and the location of the nearest chamber. The phone number is (919) 694-2948 or (919) 684-5514.

Caution!
If you suspect an embolism, place the patient on his or her left side; this will trap air in the right side of the heart.

NEAR DROWNING

Drowning accounts for 5000 deaths each year in the U.S., and is the fourth most common cause of unintentional death. Water-related accidents and deaths are closely linked to several factors, including alcohol and drug use, trauma due to boating or diving accidents, cold water, seizures, and inability to swim. Bystanders at the scene of a near drowning can often provide important history about the incident.

Aspiration of water occurs in approximately 80 percent of near drownings; in the remaining 20 percent, water is prevented from entering the lungs by laryngeal spasm. Whether aspiration occurs or not, hypoxia is the immediate mechanism of injury. Cardiac arrest—due most often to ventricular fibrillation—cerebral edema secondary to hypoxemia, and inadequate perfusion confront the first responder. If the victim is resuscitated, complications related to pulmonary damage may cause death days or weeks later.

Immediate and proper care of a near-drowning victim will often lead to a good outcome. As soon as possible, even if the victim is still being carried from the water, an airway must be established and ventilation begun. If no pulse is detected, external cardiac massage should be initiated. Supplemental oxygen is helpful. Attempts to "drain" water from the lungs are fruitless and should not be attempted. Unless trauma can be ruled out by reliable history, all near-drowning victims should be placed on a spine board and the cervical spine protected.

Accidents in cold water introduce additional variables to a resuscitation attempt. Two mechanisms operating in cold-water immersion may protect the victim, especially the child. First, the brain and heart may be protected by the "diving reflex." This adaptation shunts blood from the periphery to the central circulation and lowers the heart rate, thus offering some protection from cerebral and cardiac hypoxia. Second, hypothermia itself causes a decrease in the brain's energy requirement. These mechanisms help explain cases of survival after prolonged (30 to 40 minute) immersion in cold water. Rescuers of cold-water victims must continue resuscitation attempts until the victim is normothermic, because hypothermia mimics death so closely.

Caution!
In cold-water drownings, a declaration of death should not be considered until the victim has been warmed.

BURNS

There are approximately 2 million burn injuries per year in the United States. Perhaps 5 percent of these injuries are life-threatening; they are especially dangerous for children under 12, among whom burns are the second leading cause of death.

The organs immediately affected by burns are the skin and lungs. The immediate results of skin injury are minimal, but within a few hours fluid loss may lead to shock. If the patient is resuscitated, infection becomes a major problem in the days that follow. Inhalation injuries associated with smoky fires are usually the immediate cause of death in fires. Carbon monoxide (CO) is always present when combustion takes place and rapidly reaches toxic levels in enclosed areas. When synthetic materials (plastic, nylon, etc.) burn, other toxic fumes are produced, including cyanide, nitrous oxides, sulfur dioxides, and acids. Explosion, building collapse, and falls while trying to escape a fire may cause additional injuries and complicate the initial care of a burn victim. Unconscious victims should be treated as multiple trauma victims, with cervical spine precautions taken.

The most important aspect of field care for burn victims is removal. Extinguish burning clothing and remove the patient from the proximity of the fire. Airway, breathing, and circulation come next. Administration of high-flow oxygen by face mask helps reduce the toxicity of CO. A sterile cloth dressing soaked in cool sterile saline is often sufficient to relieve the pain of a burn.

A simple method to assess the amount of body surface area burned is the "rule of nines" (Figure 12.1). For small or patchy burns, a useful rule is that the area of the victim's palm is about 1% of total body surface area. Burns to the hands, feet, perineum, or head and neck are more serious than burns to the trunk or proximal extremities. Soot-tinged sputum, oral cavity burns, singed nasal hair, or burns around the head should alert you to the likelihood of airway damage.

Electrical burns differ markedly from thermal burns because of the pathophysiology of the injury. High-voltage electrical injury may produce local skin damage where electrical current enters and exits the victim, but the major injury will be hidden within the muscle and nerve tissue that has served as an electrical conductor. Immediate death from electrical injuries is a result of cardiac arrhythmia.

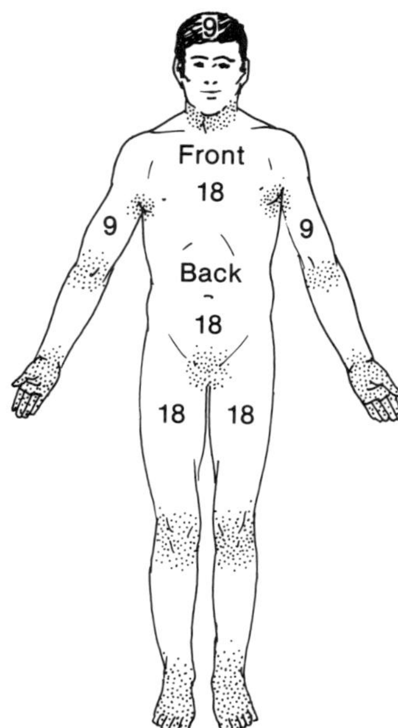

FIGURE 12.1 "Rule of nines."

Removing the patient from contact with a live electrical wire is dangerous. If power to the wire can be interrupted, this is the safest rescue method. Or, use a nonconducting object such as a dry piece of wood or a dry rope to pull or push the victim away from the wire. CPR and continuous monitoring of the cardiac rhythm during transport may be needed.

BITES

Mammalian, reptile, and spider (or arachnid) bites often require emeregency treatment. Most cases are minor, nontoxic injuries, but some are emergencies. The most pertinent information about the injury is "what" bit the patient. If it is possible to do so without endangering yourself, capture the spider or snake in question. It should be killed, but not so mangled as to prevent identification.

Spider Bites

The bites of only two species of spider native to the U.S. cause more than localized minor reaction. The black widow (*Latrodectus mactans*) is a glossy black arachnid with bright red markings on its undersurface. Classically these are shaped like an hourglass, but

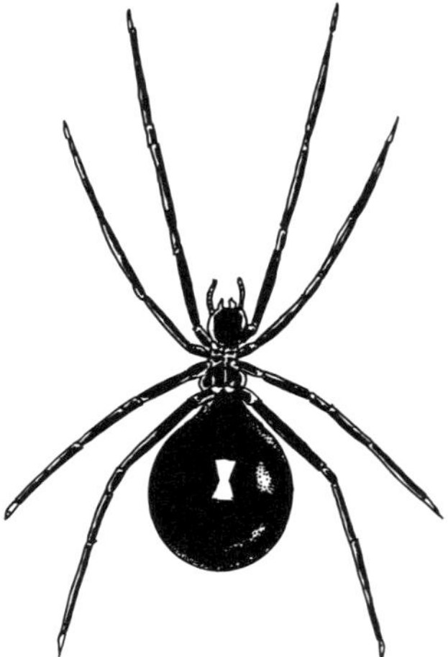

FIGURE 12.2 Black widow spider.

often they consist of two dots (Figure 12.2). The body of this spider is approximately half an inch long; including the legs, it is an inch and a half long. The black widow lives in dry, protected places such as outhouses, woodpiles, and barns. Black widow venom is a neurotoxin that initially produces a pinprick sensation at the wound site, followed soon by swelling and erythema. Within an hour, dull pain develops around the bite and spreads throughout the body. The chest and abdomen are especially affected by this pain, which may mimic an acute abdominal or cardiac pain. Nausea, vomiting, weakness, diaphoresis, and hypertension accompany the pain. Field care consists of applying an ice pack to the site and immediately transporting the victim for medical evaluation. Children and the elderly are especially at risk to suffer cardiac and respiratory dysfunction and must be carefully observed.

> **Caution!**
> The victim of a black widow bite may not link the generalized symptoms to the bite—take a good history.

The brown recluse spider (*Loxosceles reclusa*) is found primarily in the South Central U.S. and lives in woodpiles, under rocks, and often in closets. It is about an inch long including the legs, is tan or dark brown, and has a distinctive violin-shaped dark area on the dorsal head and thorax. Brown recluse bites cause pain and redness at the site, but do not progress to systemic symptoms. The bite will, however, produce a necrotic ulcer within hours. Initial care of the bite is to apply an ice pack to the area. Because of later complications, it is very important to recognize the spider and transport the patient for medical treatment (Figure 12.3).

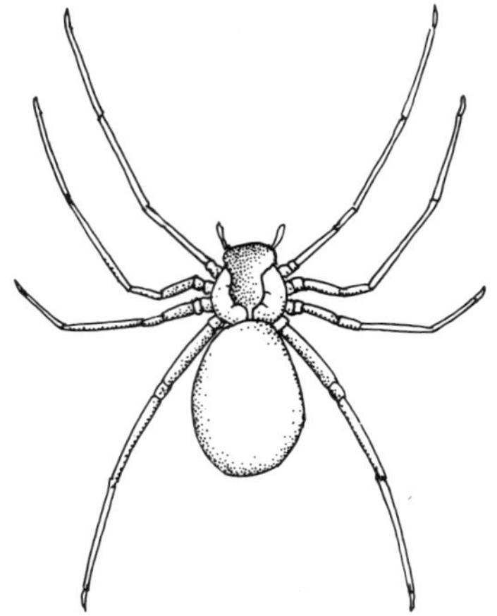

FIGURE 12.3 Brown recluse spider.

Snakebites

Venomous snakes exist in every state except Maine, Alaska, and Hawaii. Pit vipers (rattlesnakes, copperheads, water moccasins) produce 90 percent of envenomation. The coral snake, found in the coastal south and the desert Southwest, accounts for the remaining injuries. As with spiders, identification of the snake is extremely important. A triangular head, elliptical pupils, a heat-sensing pit anterior to the eye, fangs, and a single row of plates on the ventral tail are identifying characteristics of the poisonous pit viper. The colorful coral snake is easily identifed by the rhyme "Red next to yellow kills a fellow; red next to black, venom lack." It is very helpful to the physician if the offending snake can be safely killed and transported in a closed container.

Pit viper venom causes immediate and often severe pain and swelling at the site. Edema surrounding the bite gradually spreads; weakness, nausea, vomiting, fever, diaphoresis, facial numbness, muscle twitching, and hypotension commonly follow. Approximately half of pit viper bites will not produce significant envenomation. The fortunate patients will have only local symptoms of pain and will not suffer the progression of symptoms that occurs with true envenomation.

In contrast with the symptoms of pit viper bite, the symptoms caused by coral snake venom are initially minimal. The neurotoxin produces little or no pain and swelling at the site. However, within a short time the venom blocks neuromuscular transmission and muscular weakness begins. Ptosis, or drooping of the upper eyelids, is quite common, as is proximal muscle weakness, slurred speech, inability to swallow, paresthesias, vertigo, and nausea. Death occurs from respiratory arrest.

Immediate transport of the victim to a medical facility is crucial. Although various treatments for snakebites have been advocated for immediate use in the field (cut and suck, excision of the area), none of these has proven consistently effective, and all delay transport and definitive treatment. Immobilization of the patient and placing the injured part below the level of the heart is important to prevent spread of the venom. If edema is spreading in an extremity, a constricting band may be applied two to four inches above the bite. The tourniquet should be wide (at least one inch) and loose enough to permit a finger to be inserted. Do not remove the constricting band once it is applied, but loosen it at any sign of vascular compromise (decreased pulse distally or decreased capillary refill at the nail beds).

Caution!
If swelling advances above the tourniquet, apply a second tourniquet higher on the extremity.

Dogs and Cat Bites

An estimated 2 million animals bites occur annually in the U.S., and dogs account for 80 percent or more of these. Cats are responsible for up to 15 percent of bite injuries. The severity of a bite injury results from mechanical tearing of the tissue. Thus, the larger the attacking animal, the greater the potential injury. Bites from large animals can cause hemorrhage, airway damage, penetration of body cavities (chest, abdomen, skull). The animal can cause blunt trauma by striking the victim or causing the victim to fall as he attempts to escape. Small animals cause minor laceration or puncture wounds. All bite wounds are contaminated and very likely to become infected.

Initial treament of animal bites may be as uncomplicated as a simple dressing for small wounds or as complex as fluid resuscitation and airway control for a severely injured victim. Cervical spine injury is possible in some instances and must be considered. History, as always, is most helpful. Was the animal domestic or wild? If domestic, was it vaccinated? Was the attack provoked or unprovoked? Did the animal appear ill? If the animal cannot be captured, the answers to these questions may help guide the physician in deciding to treat for rabies. You can offer some reassurance to the victim concerning rabies: Squirrels, rodents, cattle, horses, and pigs almost never transmit this disease.

THERMAL STRESS

Cold Injury

Exposure to cold may cause frostbite and associated near-freezing injuries when a localized area of the body is affected, or hypothermia when body temperature is lowered. Cold injuries are increasing as more people participate in outdoor recreation, and hypothermia is increasingly recognized as a significant problem in the elderly and debilitated.

Chilblain and trench foot (or immersion foot) are localized nonfreezing injuries that result from prolonged exposure of skin to cold or cold water. Neither of these injuries commonly presents for field care, but the more severe freezing injury, frostbite, often does. A decrease in air temperature can be augmented by exposure to wetness or by the chilling effect of wind. Both of these mechanisms can dramatically increase the amount of heat lost from an exposed or underinsulated body part. Commonly, appendages such as fingers, toes, nose, and ears are frostbitten. These body parts have less vascular supply than the more proximal areas, and in a cold environment vasoconstriction often occurs in these areas as a heat-saving mechanism. As tissue temperature decreases, ice crystals begin to form in the tissue and cells are damaged. Intensive vasoconstriction accompanies this freezing and the part becomes even cooler.

A frostbitten part presents as white nonblanching tissue that is soft when compressed if the injury is superficial (that is, affecting skin and subcutaneous tissue only). If the frostbite injury is deep, the tissue is hard and feels woody when compressed. Frostbitten areas are usually numb before treatment and do not show capillary refill when compressed. Rapid rewarming is the immediate treatment. A water bath of between 100 and 112 degrees F will reverse tissue freezing in about 30 minutes. Therefore, rewarming should not be attempted without adequate facilities. In rescue situations, it is preferable to cover the injured area with a soft dressing to prevent blunt injury and transport the patient to a hospital.

Caution!
Partial thawing followed by reexposure to cold is more destructive to tissue than keeping the tissue frozen until facilities are available to thaw the part and keep it warm.

Hypothermia

Hypothermia is a decrease in body core temperature, most readily measured as rectal temperature, below 35 °C (95 °F). Exposure to cold water and cold air is an obvious cause. The elderly or debilitated person who lives in a cold house or is improperly dressed during cold weather can also become hypothermic. Surveys have demonstrated that hypothermia affects 10 percent of the elderly. Severity of symptoms increases as body core temperature decreases. Mild hypothermia (33–35 °C, 92–95 °F) causes apathy, forgetfulness, uncoordination, poor judgment, decreased communication, slurred speech, and ataxia. "Paradoxical undressing" may occur: the victim removes clothing even while becoming colder. As body core temperature decreases further, the level of consciousness decreases from stupor to frank coma with absence of response to all stimuli. Pulse and respiration decrease and may not be detectable; pupils dilate and become nonreactive. A cardiac monitor attached to the patient will often show a range of dysrhythmias, ranging from atrial fibrillation to asystole. The cool heart is particularly susceptible to ventricular fibrillation. The skin is cool and dry because circulation has been shunted from the skin to the core organs.

Initial care of hypothermia is complicated. Inappropriate management may lead to life-threatening cardiac problems. The cold heart is very irritable, and stresses such as CPR or rough patient handling can precipitate dysrhythmia, most commonly ventricular fibrillation. Field treatment of responsive patients consists of recognizing the problem, covering the patient with blankets, removing wet clothing, and transporting the victim. The unresponsive hypothermia victim must be assessed like any other unresponsive patient, with certain cautions. If there are no respirations, ventilation should be started. The search for pulses or heart tones should be thorough, because these are often barely perceptible. If no cardiac activity is detected, external cardiac massage should be started. If any cardiac activity is noted, no compressions should be done. Administration of heated, humidified oxygen can add heat to the core. Careful and gentle handling is essential. Severe hypothermia is often indistinguishable from death. Hypothermic victims should be aggressively resuscitated, and resuscitation should continue until the patient is "warm and dead." Remarkable recoveries have occurred after prolonged resuscitation.

Hyperthermia (Heat Illness)

When the body is unable to dispose of excess heat, the body temperature rises. Heat stresses commonly affect young or active people who work and exercise in warm environments. But, just as with hypothermia, the elderly and debilitated may suffer heat illness simply by living in a warm, poorly ventilated apartment.

The body regulates temperature accurately and maintains a constant temperature of approximately 37 °C (98.6 °F) by releasing heat when there is an excess. When air temperature is less than body temperature, radiation of heat from the body accomplishes about 65 percent of necessary heat loss; water vaporization by lungs and skin accounts for additional heat losses. However, at air temperatures above 37 °C, heat is lost primarily by sweating—vaporization of water at the skin surface by the body's heat. As relative humidity increases the efficiency of sweating decreases, and at 90 to 95 percent relative humidity there is minimal heat loss from sweating. The combination of warm air temperature and high humidity is responsible for heat illness, especially when the body produces excess heat (muscle activity) or has reduced heat reduction ability (as is the case in the elderly or chronically ill). Dehydration also limits the body's ability to dissipate heat by sweating, and predisposes individuals to heat illness.

Minor heat syndromes, such as heat edema, heat syncope, and heat cramps, occur from heat exposure without an increase in body temperature. These are self-limited illnesses that respond quickly to a cool environment and rehydration. Heat stroke, the deadly form of heat illness, is characterized by an increase in body temperature (usually above 40 °C, or 104 °F). *Exertional heat stroke* affects young, fit persons who stress themselves in heat and humidity. Military recruits, joggers, and football players are at risk, especially when unacclimated to the heat. Inability to concentrate, decreased sweating, headache, nausea, and lightheadedness usually precede bizarre behavior, confusion, seizures, and coma. The patient will feel hot and is usually sweating. *Classic heat stroke* affects the elderly, debilitated, and very young. It develops over a few days, rather than in a few hours, as in exertional heat stroke. A warm environment and inadequate fluid intake lead to dehydration, headache, and dizziness and progress to confusion and coma. There is sometimes an absence of sweating due to dehydration. Heat stroke victims exhibit tachycardia, hyperventilation, hypotension, an elevated temperature, and an altered mental state.

Rapid cooling should begin at once in suspected heat stroke victims. Undress and place the patient in the coolest available environment (shade, air-conditioned truck). Apply water to the victim's skin and, if a fan is available, blow air over the exposed wet skin to hasten evaporation. Ice packs may be applied to the groin or axilla. Airway protection and respiratory support may be necessary.

RADIATION AND HAZARDOUS MATERIALS

Potentially lethal chemicals and radioactive material are transported daily in our country. Nuclear power plants and industrial facilities store these materials in all parts of the U.S. An incident involving hazardous materials or radioactivity is ever-present.

Caution!
Planning and preparation is essential in handling incidents involving hazardous material and radioactivity.

Initial management of a radioactive or chemical exposure requires knowledge of (1) the material involved and its toxicity; (2) methods of handling the patient that will not expose the rescuer to injury or contamination; (3) treatment of immediately life-threatening injuries in a safe manner; and (4) initial decontamination of the victim, if necessary. A discussion of the large number of chemicals and radiation sources now present in our environment is beyond the scope of this volume. However, a rescuer unfamiliar with a hazardous material or radiation source should seek help at once from an authority such as the U.S. Department of Energy Regional Coordinating Office or a local resource person (often a fire department official or industrial safety officer). Nonetheless, some generalizations can be made about hazardous materials and radioactive substances. Distance from the source provides safety. Toxic fumes are diluted in the open atmosphere, and the energy of radioactive emissions decreases with distance and shielding. Removal or dilution of a toxic substance will decrease injury. Removing contaminated clothes and diluting the chemical with water will often prevent further injury. Protective clothing and a self-contained breathing apparatus must be used in many situations. Local advisers should be identified and available when the need arises. Specialized training and proper equipment should be available for rescuers called upon in an emergency involving hazardous material.

CONCLUSION

The environment may both cause injury and interfere with emergency medical care. There is a difference between rendering aid on a bright spring afternoon and struggling with a near-drowning victim stuck under an ice floe in a blizzard. Trauma care is challenging under the best of circumstances. The environment is a very real factor in determining how a patient can be managed. The physician awaiting the patient's arrival in a well-equipped and comfortable emergency unit may not appreciate the adversity under which you work. Always do what is safe for yourself and best for the patient.

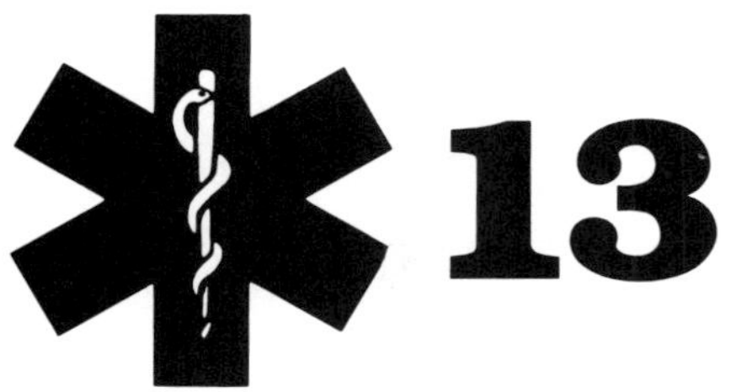

13

Extrication, Packaging, and Transport

INTRODUCTION

Extrication can be the most physically and mentally challenging situation you face. Many EMTs receive only minimal instruction in extrication procedures, and find themselves in situations for which they are poorly prepared. No training or review manual can serve as an acceptable substitute for an organized, field-oriented vehicle rescue training program. The purpose of this chapter is to outline some of the basic considerations of functioning at the scene of a crash, and to define your responsiblities for managing these incidents. Rapid assessment of the patient both during and after extrication is a basic yet important skill. Having made this evaluation, you must prepare the victim for evacuation (usually by ground or air) to an appropriate medical facility for definitive treatment. To insure the health and safety of both patient and care-giver, you must package the victim to prevent further injury, accommodate changes in the patient's condition, and safeguard the rescue team.

OBJECTIVES

At the completion of this chapter, you should be able to:

1. Explain the importance of protective equipment for rescue workers.
2. Describe the ten phases of a systematic rescue.

3. Describe the use of accident scene assessment to manage vehicle rescue decision making.
4. Define the wide variety of rescue equipment available to the rescuer.
5. Describe the primary objectives of packaging patients.
6. List the phases of the pretransport and transport process and describe their value.
7. State your responsibility during patient transport and define the components of an ambulance-to-hospital report.
8. Explain how to complete patient transfer at the hospital.

EXTRICATION

Your role in vehicle rescue incidents will tend to be location- and situation-specific. An EMT working in an urban EMS system is generally held more responsible for emergency care than for rescue. Upon receipt of a call that is likely to involve extrication of trapped victims, many areas utilize a tiered incident-response system that simultaneously dispatches EMS, fire, rescue, and law enforcement personnel. Rural and suburban areas may not have such resources, in which case emergency units are self-contained and equipped to handle both medical and rescue needs. It is your responsibility to ascertain your role in local operations, and to adapt training and proficiency regimens to fulfill these mission requirements.

Protective Equipment

Emergency personnel working in or around extrication operations must wear protective equipment. EMS workers tend to aggressively protect victims but neglect themselves. Sharp metal shards, broken glass, and spilled fuel are but a few of the common hazards encountered at rescue scenes. To avoid injury, wear equipment that will protect the (1) head and eyes, (2) hands, (3) body (torso), (4) feet, and (5) respiratory system.

Caution!
The hazards to rescuers are no less than those that threaten victims.

Head and Eyes. Be especially careful to protect your head and eyes during rescue operations. Many extrication procedures produce flying debris and particles that can quickly injure or incapacitate crew members. Add preexisting conditions, such as downed electric lines or fire, and the need for such protection becomes obvious. A fire-fighter's helmet with face shield, coupled with a pair of wrap-around safety goggles (or glasses), provides excellent protection from the majority of hazards you will encounter.

Caution!
An incapacitated rescuer is of no help to the victim—protect yourself so you can help others.

Hands. Your hands are fundamental to effective field operations. For extrication operations, fire-fighter's gloves or medium-weight leather gloves work well. Some newer models include puncture-and-cut-resistant liners (usually Kevlar), which enhance protection. Avoid thin leather or cloth athletic gloves, as most fail to offer the hazard resistance needed for the extrication environment.

Body. A fire-fighter's turnout coat is a good choice for protecting the torso and arms. There are also several types of "EMS jackets" on the market that appear well suited to crash rescue. Besides providing some degree of impact protection, these garments are resistant to many chemicals and are water-repellent. In cooler climates, supplemental liners can be added to provide warmth. Whatever you use, know its *limitations!*

Feet. Safety shoes or bunker boots (fire-fighter's boots) are the best choice. Steel shanks and toe guards add extra protection. Low-cut uniform shoes or leather tennis shoes are inadequate.

Respiratory Protection. Though you may need it only occasionally, you should be competent with the use of self-contained breathing apparatus. Many vehicular components produce highly toxic gases when burned or even heated. Even short-term exposure can produce lasting medical impairments. The key is to be trained and certified in the use of these devices *before* you need them. The rescue scene is not the best classroom!

Phases of Extrication

Extrication has been described as a "system of operations." In fact, it is a system within a system. The basic theory of vehicle crash rescue was established in the mid-1970s. The system consists of 11 steps or phases:

1. readiness
2. response
3. assessment
4. hazard control
5. support operations
6. gaining access
7. emergency care
8. disentanglement
9. removal and transfer
10. termination

Readiness. To work safely and competently in the extrication setting, you must be physically and mentally prepared. Vehicle technology and materials change constantly. To maintain readiness, you must constantly train *and* retrain with the available equipment, and that equipment must be meticulously maintained.

Caution!
The lives of both victims and rescuer depend on equipment that is well maintained and functioning properly.

Response. This phase spans the time from the initial call for help until the arrival of the rescue unit at the scene. Be aware of factors that can affect response: weather, time of day, road conditions, traffic congestion, and crowding from local factories, churches, and schools. Oddly enough, this phase also seems among the most hazardous, for the majority of EMS crashes (and injuries) occur *before* the unit ever reaches the scene. The rescue site (on the road, over a cliff, submerged in water) dictates the complexity and type of effort needed to reach victims.

Scene Assessment. Very similar to the "size-up" procedures used by fire-fighters, the assessment phase is the time to match incident requirements against available capabilities and resources. This initial assessment should be conducted by the crew member most competent in rescue operations, regardless of rank.

Caution!
Do not allow tunnel vision (or an overzealous desire to help) to influence the critical process of incident decision making.

In vehicle rescue, there are two pressing questions:

1. Are there injured persons?
2. Are other persons or property endangered?

From these two questions, you can formulate the strategies and evaluate the resources you will need to manage the incident scene. As additional data are gathered, you can make more detailed decisions involving allocation of patients, personnel, and equipment. Typically, four primary points are examined:

Number and types of vehicles involved. From an incident management standpoint, there is a great deal of difference between a school bus incident and a single-vehicle mishap. To reach intelligent, workable decisions on how to allocate resources, you must pay particular attention to the magnitude of the crash scene, as it will frequently influence or even mandate a given EMS response.

Number of victims and nature of injuries. With the advent of trauma care systems, patient allocation and destination decisions have now become more patient-oriented. If patients are critically injured, transporting them to the closest facility is a failed concept. You must obtain accurate patient information, since it will directly affect not only where a patient is taken, but how the patient is transported. Match the regional hospital resources to the needs of the patient.

Hazard Control. Traffic, unstable vehicles, spilled fuel, and many other potentially harmful circumstances are frequently present at rescue sites. Before patient care *or* extrication activities can begin, each of these hazards must be eliminated or controlled. Based on prevailing conditions and the information gathered during assessment, various hazards must be resolved on the priority of threat (or potential threat) to rescuers and patients alike.

Support Operations. Conditions at the crash site are not always conducive to easy rescue. Weather and darkness require protection, shelter and illumination. Spectators may unintentionally interfere with rescue operations and place themselves in jeopardy. Crowd control is mandatory. Preservation of the scene is necessary, especially if foul play or a fatality has occurred.

Gaining Access. During this phase, emergency personnel either utilize existing openings or make new openings in order to reach victims. In motor vehicle extrication, usual routes of entry include doors, windows, and the body of the vehicle.

Emergency Care. Once you reach the patient, begin emergency care and patient protection. This phase continues until the patient arrives at the hospital.

Disentanglement. This involves removing entrapment mechanisms from the victim. This is generally accomplished through widening of existing or new openings and/or forcible removal of vehicle components or debris from around the victim.

Removal and Transfer. This phase consists of moving the victim to the waiting stretcher and transporting him or her by ambulance or air rescue to a medical facility. In most vehicle crashes, the victim will require packaging prior to transport. This applies for both ground and air evacuation. There are three fundamental considerations in packaging. Let's briefly consider each.

Equipment Commonly Used

As stated earlier, a review manual cannot replace comprehensive drills in vehicle rescue procedures. EMTs should learn the many types of equipment, from screwdrivers to complex hydraulic equipment used in extrication operations. Availability of this equipment and protocol for its use will vary from area to area, but you should know not only what tools are available, but also how (and why) a given tool is used. Figures 13.1–13.6 illustrate some of the major types of equipment used in vehicle rescue.

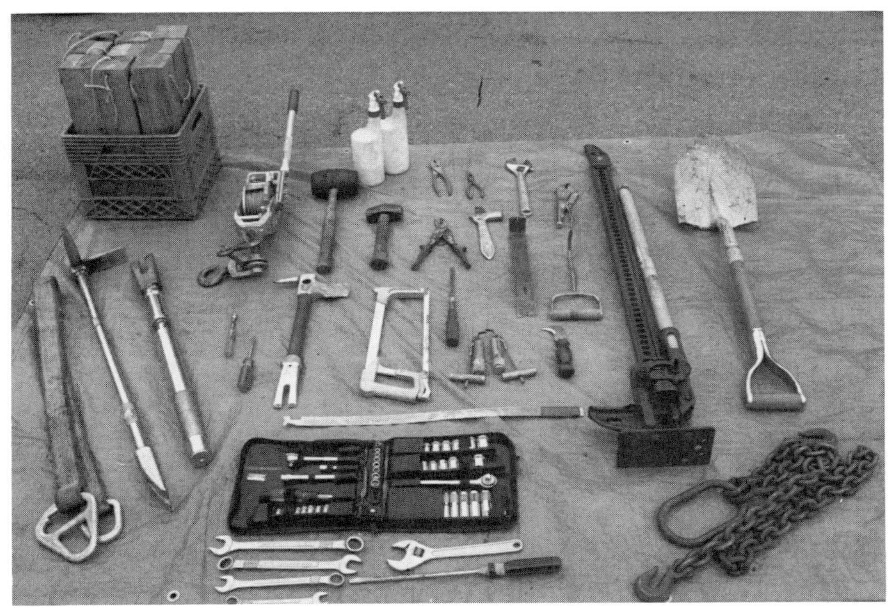

FIGURE 13.1 Hand tools.

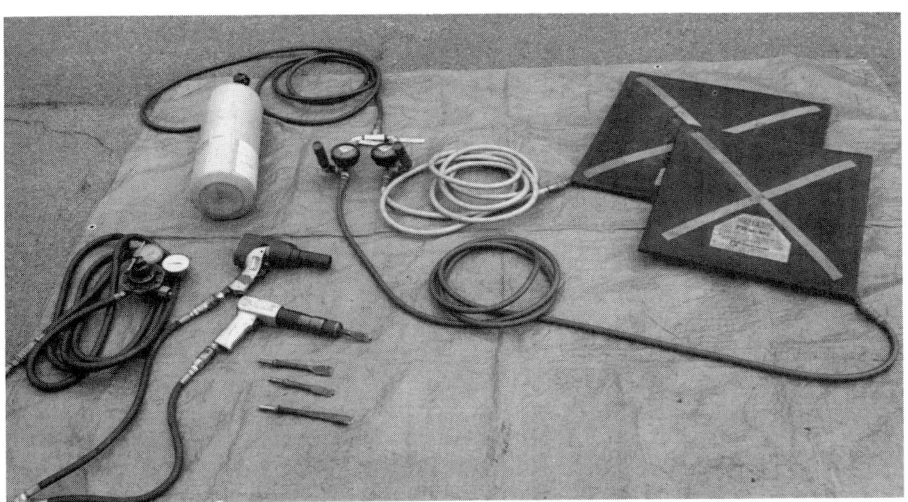

FIGURE 13.2 Air-powered tools.

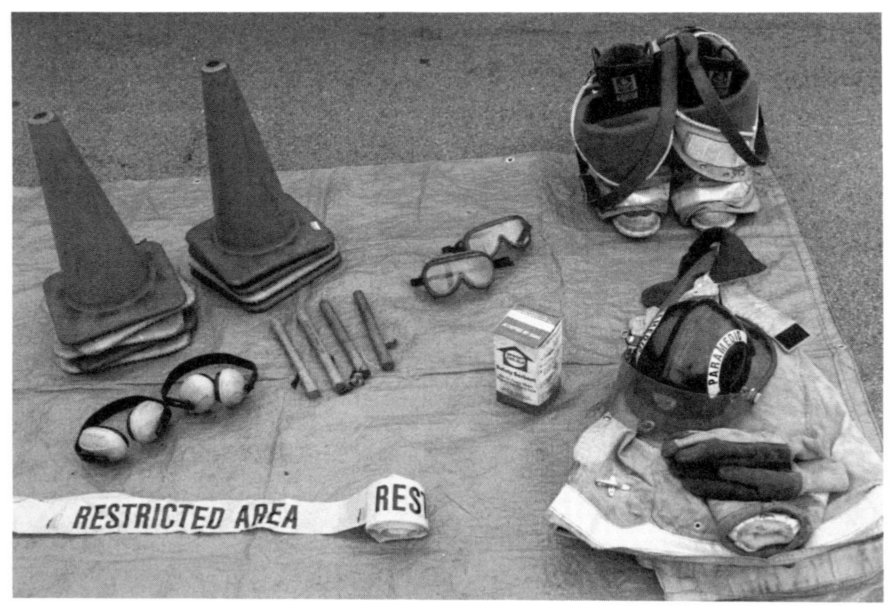

FIGURE 13.3 Hazard control equipment.

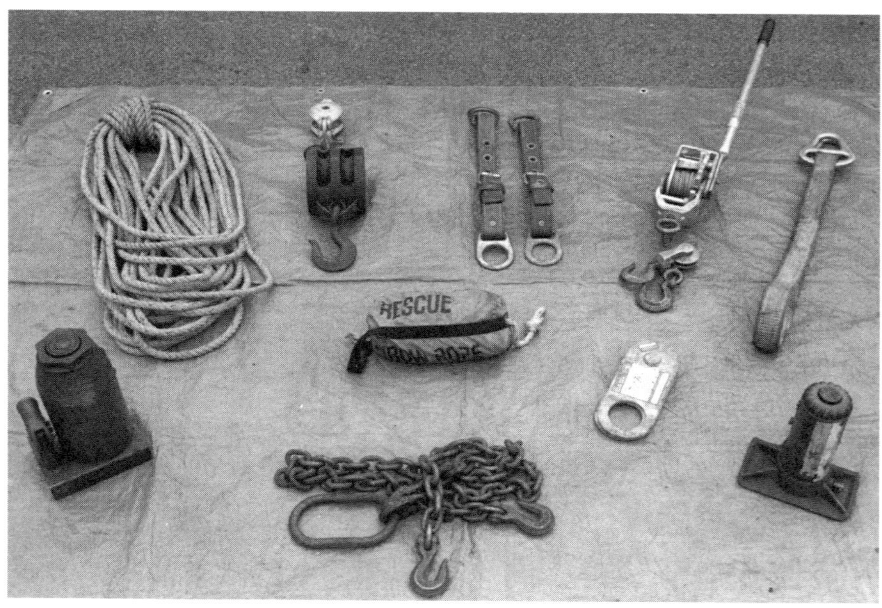

FIGURE 13.4 Lifting and pulling devices.

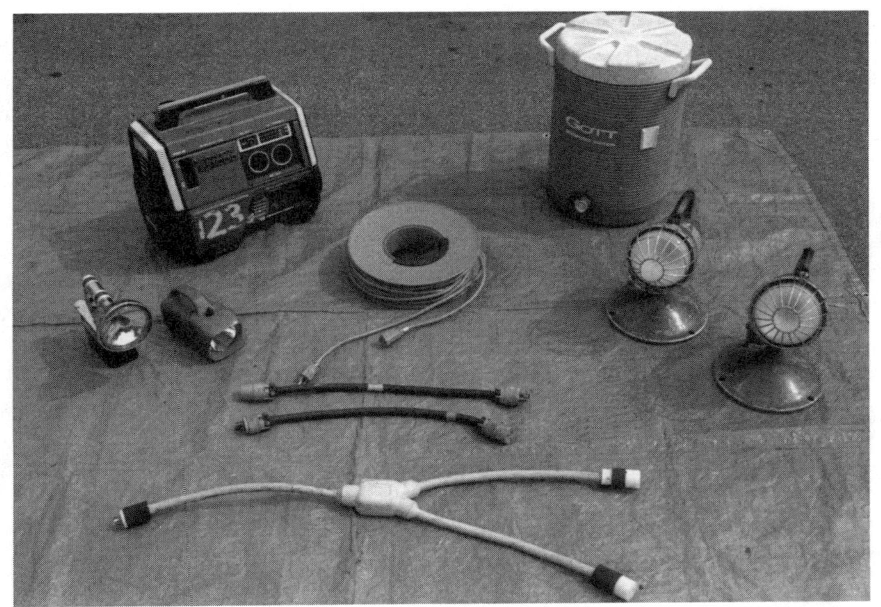

FIGURE 13.5 Support equipment.

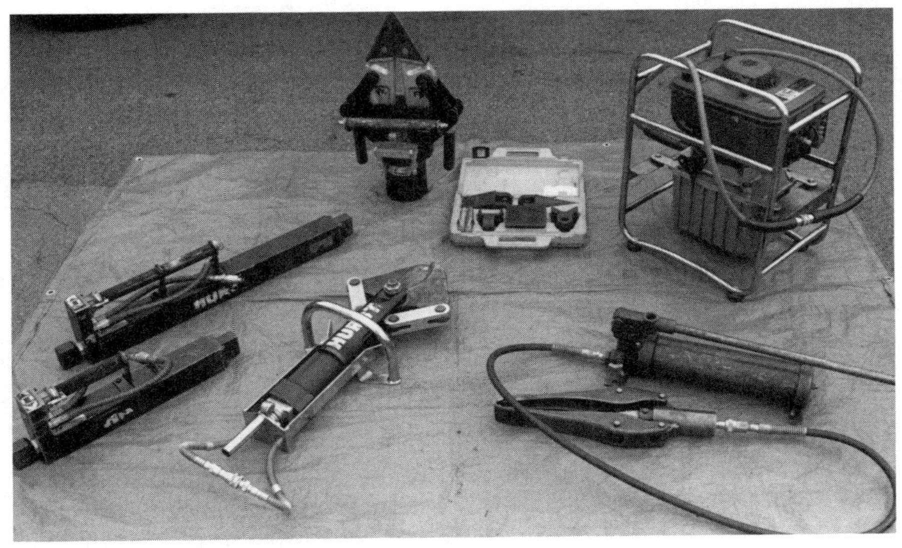

FIGURE 13.6 Hydraulic equipment.

Prevention of Further Injury or the Aggravation of Existing Injury

Care of the trauma patient presents the emergency medical technician with the unique situation of practicing a form of preventative medicine *after* an insult has occurred. In many cases, actions taken (or not taken) by the EMT will directly benefit or jeopardize a patient's recovery. Therefore, EMTs must be able to utilize the packaging equipment at their disposal to move the victim safely, regardless of scene conditions. In trauma victims, *packaging* generally indicates spinal immobilization, coupled with other immobilization devices for managing the conditions generated by the patient, his or her injuries, the environment, and the method of transport.

Placement of Patient to Accommodate Changes in Condition

Providing emergency care would be much less stressful if "stabalized" victims were incapable of developing radical changes in their condition. This, of course, is fantasy. The EMT must anticipate and accommodate these changes. Rapid intervention to prevent aspiration, shock, or other life-threatening changes in patient status are often necessary. Careful planning for these contingencies during the packaging process will help you respond to patient needs without worsening existing injuries.

Safety of Patients and Crew Members

Trauma often occurs in hostile environments. Transportation mishaps, household or farm injuries, and encounters with hazardous materials are but a few of the more common settings.

To an injured, disoriented patient, the ambulance is probably a hostile environment as well. The EMT must realize this. Trauma victims sacrifice much of their ability to control their environment. Careful packaging helps reassure the patient that active measures are being taken to insure a safe transition to definitive treatment.

Patient care is always a primary concern, but protection of emergency personnel is equally important. Efficient, effective packaging helps preclude the possibility of injury from a combative patient or the "patient missile" that can occur with emergency stops.

Caution!
Careful packaging is similar to insurance: Both work on the assumption that disaster will not occur, but protect the patient and the rescuer just in case.

Termination. Also known as *recovery*, this phase entails all post incident activity required to secure personnel and equipment, and return them to duty-read status.

TRANSPORT

There was a time when transport consisted of little more than placing the victim on a stretcher and speeding to the nearest hospital. Advances in training, technology, and pubic awareness of EMS systems have made this process more complex. Patient transport includes three phases: (1) pretransport, (2) transfer, and (3) posttransport.

Pretransport Activities

As the transporting EMT, you should "check the work" before the unit moves. Too often, excellent packaging is compromised by unsafe patient placement in the emergency unit. Therefore, pay careful attention to checking patient-related equipment, quickly rechecking the patient, and securing personal effects. After placing the patient in the emergency unit, always check the stretcher. Loading often presents the possibility of a less-than-adequate lock-in of the cot. Carefully inspect the locking mechanisms (cot wall rails, center mounts, etc.) to insure adequate latching. Few events in the ambulance are as calamitous as a "runaway cot." The cot and patient become a "missile," with the likely target the EMT. Such mishaps quickly degrade patient confidence and can aggravate existing problems or create new injuries.

Straps also need adjustment. EMS providers use straps for many purposes, such as patient immobilization or securing equipment. Unfortunately, straps tend to work loose as patients and equipment are moved to the unit. Be sure all straps are properly adjusted before moving the unit. Loose equipment or, worse, a loose patient will quickly compromise your ability to continue patient care. In more extreme situations, such as a combative patient or emergency driving maneuvers, improperly secured patients or equipment may become life-threatening hazards.

Inflatable patient-care equipment also benefits from a quick check. The PASG, air splints, and vacuum splinting devices are frequently exposed to metal fragments, broken glass, and other harmful debris. Over time, small leaks develop and inflation valves wear out. Even with frequent inspection, it is not uncommon for these devices to fail when placed on a patient. Palpate each compartment of these devices to ensure proper inflation. Also inspect the valves, resolving signs of obstruction or leakage. If you cannot readjust or reinflate the device, consider changing to another set before moving the unit.

Airways, oxygen masks, splints, and bandages also benefit from a quick inspection. Look for proper fit, flow rates, good positioning, and proper operation. Extra effort on the "front end" can often preclude disaster later on.

Transfer Activities. Immediate transport is indicated for most seriously injured patients. Further assessment is done en route to the hospital. Next, perform a quick yet thorough patient exam. Attention to seemingly small details can make the trip less physically and psychologically demanding for both you and the patient. Obtain a baseline appraisal of the patient's status just before leaving the scene. This information will allow you to detect subtle (yet often significant) changes before more dramatic consequences occur. This exam should concentrate on airway and ventilation, circulation, vital signs, comfort, and psychological support.

Airway and ventilation. A patient's condition rarely remains static throughout transfer. It usually improves or declines. A common source of compromise is the patient's airway and respiratory status. Maintenance of a patent airway is always a priority. Because trauma victims are prone to develop airway problems, vomitus, blood, body secretions, or foreign material must be anticipated. To cope with these problems, you can use four universally available tools: the senses of sight, sound, smell, and touch.

Sight: Observe the patient's position on the stretcher. In some instances, repositioning can help the patient exchange air more easily. Repositioning, though, should not be undertaken if contraindicated by other problems. If immobilized on a spine board, the patient may be rotated onto the left side, provided he or she can be moved as a unit. Once the patient and board are in place, pad behind the board with pillows or blankets and firmly secure the board with straps.

Observe the patient's face, neck, and chest. Carefully note skin color and condition. Especially watch for signs of cyanosis or pallor, and note the presence (or absence) of perspiration. Check the trachea and neck veins. If you note a shift from midline (trachea) or distention (neck veins), suspect a tension pneumothorax or cardiac tamponade.

Observe how the patient breathes. Are the chest muscles retracting? If so, is the movement equal on both sides? Look for obvious bruising and/or flail segments.

Sound: Listen carefully for respiratory sounds that seem abnormal. In trauma victims, snoring or low-pitched sounds frequently accompany soft-tissue injuries or obstructions. Bubbling or gurgling usually indicates foreign material or obstructions from vomitus, blood, secretions, or, occasionally, pulmonary edema. High-pitched sounds, such as "crowing" or stridor, can be signs of laryngospasm or upper respiratory obstruction. Wheezing may indicate a mechanical obstruction of the lower airway.

Touch: Note the condition of the skin. Is it hot, cool, dry, or damp? Feel for crepitus in the chest and neck. Palpate the trachea to determine midline placement.

Smell: Odor—often overlooked but possibly very important—can provide pertinent information during assessment. Note the aroma of alcohol, acetone, or other unusual smells.

Remember that trauma patients often require active intervention to maintain respiratory integrity. Suction, insertion of airways, and ventilatory assistance will often be required. Be sure the patient is placed in a manner that accommodates these procedures. Have support equipment (face masks, bag-valve-masks, airways, suction, demand valves) ready.

Circulation. Check for a carotid and a radial pulse. If a carotid pulse is absent, initiate CPR according to local protocol. If the carotid pulse is present, but both radial pulses are absent, suspect shock and administer appropriate interventions.

Quickly examine splints and bandages for the possible need for strengthening, loosening, or tightening. Check distal circulation and sensation before and after adjustments are made. Watch for blood loss into bandages, splints, or bedding. It is not uncommon for formerly adequate bleeding controls to be compromised during transfer. If bandaging materials become blood-soaked, add more dressing and pressure to the dressing and maintain elevation of the injured extremity.

Vital signs. To adequately assess patient status during field assessment, emergency medical care, and transfer, it is important to obtain serial vital signs. Too often, EMT assessments of "stable" vital signs are based on the one set of vital signs recorded during secondary assessment. Never assume a patient is stable based on a single set of findings.

Take the time to obtain a set of vital signs—including pulse, respiration, blood pressure, level of consciousness, and pupillary response—just before moving the ambulance. This set may become very important, as it is frequently impossible to obtain reliable measurements once you are moving.

Comfort and psychological support. Remember that patients usually view the inside of an ambulance as an unfamiliar environment. Common sense indicates that comfortable patients will be much easier to manage than victims who feel they have been placed in an uncomfortable position. Talk to patients, reassure them that they are being well cared for, and ask what you can do to make them more comfortable. If possible, pad straps, rigid contact points, and splints. Take a little extra time to blouse (infold) sheets and blankets. During inclement weather, use plastic sheets or disposable blankets to protect the patient from the elements.

The minimal time and effort expended for psychological support can create a lasting positive impression of your efforts to the patient and family. Such actions demonstrate your concern and show that you are not simply putting in your time.

Transfer usually lends no significant positive effects on the patient's condition. Consequently, you must continue life support measures and patient monitoring en route. Pay special attention to maintenance of a patient airway.

Watch closely for changes in the patient's condition. Vital signs should be obtained at frequent intervals throughout the transfer. Changes in blood pressure, level of consciousness, or respiratory status may signal important trends in patient status.

Record pertinent findings on the run sheet and report them to the hospital.

The ambulance crew must function as a team, particularly when transporting trauma patients. Motion inside the patient compartment can aggravate patient injuries, as well as your ability to provide care. The driver must be aware of changes in patient status, particularly if the changes indicate a change from routine to emergency mode. To obtain the "ride" needed, you must keep the driver informed. You must also be able to provide concise radio reports to receiving hospitals. Accurate reporting allows the medical facility to arrange its resources to meet the special requirements of each patient, and alleviates the problems created when a trauma victim arrives unannounced. Individual formats may differ by locale, but the following information is pertinent to any report:

1. Identify the hospital.
2. Identify your unit.
3. Identify yourself and your level of training.
4. Briefly describe what has happened.
5. Present pertinent background information.
6. Present findings from the patient exam.
7. Report suspected injuries or conditions.
8. Explain what emergency medical care has been given.
9. Give estimated arrival time.

Prior to arrival at the hospital, monitor airway and vital signs and pay particular attention to bandages and splints. Check skin color, distal circulation, and sensation frequently. Watch carefully for blood-soaked bandages. A significant volume of blood can pool in stretcher linen without becoming obvious. Remember to add dressing and bandaging material to existing compresses rather than replacing them.

Posttransport Activities

Upon arriving at the hospital, try to minimize interruption in care. The transfer of patient care responsibility must not be haphazard. An orderly transition helps insure that the needs of the patient, the EMS staff, and hospital personnel are all accommodated. Such a transition involves securing the patient and securing the crew and unit.

Secure the patient. Unless advised by radio, you must first ascertain just where the patient is to be taken. Once in the treatment area, assist the hospital staff in moving the patient onto the hospital stretcher. Frequently, the hospital staff may ask you to stand by and assist with patient care and equipment management.

After responsibility for patient care is assumed by the medical facility, an appropriate staff member (usually a physician or nurse) should be given a brief update on the patient. Include any relevant observations, especially major changes in vital signs or level of consciousness. If possible, submit a copy of the ambulance run sheet to the staff member.

Don't forget the patient's personal effects, or accompanying family and friends. Direct nonpatients to appropriate reception areas. This assists the hospital in maintaining order and usually hastens the completion of necessary paperwork. If personal effects were transported, obtain a signed release before turning them over to the family or the facility.

Caution!
EMS personnel may be accused of property theft if personal articles are missing. Protect yourself by obtaining a property release from family or hospital.

Secure the Unit and the Crew. After the patient is received by the hospital, your efforts generally turn towards return to service. Compilation of concise medical records and run reports is a necessity. If possible, allow a few minutes for "decompression" following a stressful call. This allows the crew to return to "normalcy" and think through their actions and reactions without the hindrance of an adrenaline "rush." Each crew member should have input into response records to assure continuity. This helps prevent situations where one crew member is forced to speculate about the actions of another.

Sanitation has also become a major concern. Emergency personnel must exercise extreme caution in dealing with body fluids. "Glove up" for every patient. In some cases, masks and even goggles should be strongly considered. If skin surfaces do become contaminated, wash the areas thoroughly with an approved germicidal/virocidal cleanser. For unit and equipment sanitation, use 1:10 solution of chlorine bleach and water.

> **Caution!**
> Trauma is a time-sensitive problem. The principles outlined in this chapter are important to the safe and orderly handling of the patient. In the bleeding, unstable patient, omission of certain steps may be necessary.

CONCLUSION

Extrication, packaging, and transport are indelibly linked with the EMT. The first rule of trauma care is "do no further harm." Yet much harm can come to the patient if transport is necessarily delayed or the patient is further endangered by unsafe practices. The principles described in this chapter provide the underpinnings for sound decision making in the field.

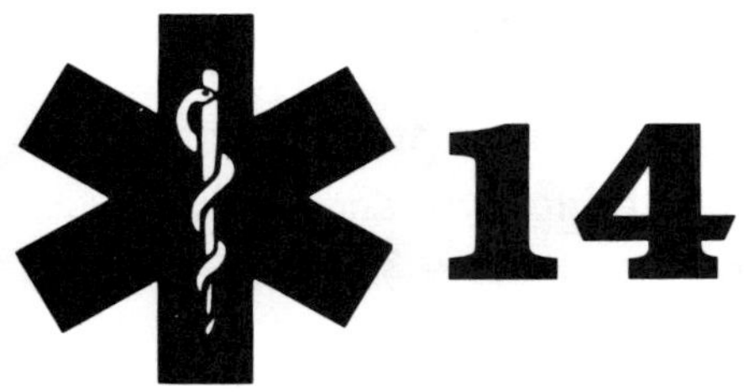

Special Problems in Field Trauma Management

INTRODUCTION

Trauma does not always occur on a well-lighted highway just a few miles from a trauma center. Some of the more challenging problems to the EMT occur when trauma is sustained in a remote or hostile environment or when the number of casualties exceeds the capabilities to care for them. This chapter considers special problems in trauma care, including water rescue, farm injuries, cave and mine rescue, mass casualties, and airplane crashes. The thread tying these problems together is the need for a plan. There is no substitute for preparation. Special problems require special planning and special equipment.

OBJECTIVES

At the completion of this chapter, you should be able to:

1. Describe what happens to a victim of impending submersion.
2. Evaluate the risk–benefit factor in providing water rescue, and describe measures to enhance safety for the rescuer.
3. Describe the technique used for the face-down victim and how to safely transport the victim out of the water.
4. Define the relationship between water temperature and survival for both victim and rescuer.

5. Relate the factors that predispose to farm-related injuries.
6. Describe the special problems related to farm accidents.
7. Distinguish between the three types of mining operations in the U.S. and recognize hazards created by each.
8. Define the EMT's responsibility at mine accidents.
9. Describe the special equipment needed during cave rescue.
10. List the principle hazards of cave rescue and how they can be avoided.
11. Explain what agencies need to be represented on a community-wide disaster committee.
12. Define the responsibilities of a disaster committee.
13. Define the six principles of disaster management and their command officers.
14. Describe the areas of responsibility for noncommand officers.
15. List five types of disaster drills and describe their educational objectives.
16. Explain how to critique a disaster drill.
17. Identify the weakest part of a disaster plan and list ways to correct the weakness.
18. Summarize the principles of general aviation safety, aircraft structure, components of emergency operations, and common aircraft hazards.
19. Define reporting and dispatching criteria for missing aircraft and aircraft crashes.
20. Describe safe-approach guidelines for aircraft accidents.
21. Review aircraft fire-rescue guidelines, techniques, and equipment.
22. Explain principles of crash investigation and scene preservation.
23. Instruct personnel in the handling of water crashes, crashes into buildings, and witnessed helicopter crashes.

WATER RESCUE

Nearly two-thirds of the earth is covered by water. Oceans, lakes, rivers, ponds, and, of course, swimming pools present a constant threat for water-related trauma and/or near drowning. Therefore, you will sometimes be called upon to care for a victim of water-related injuries. In both the United States and Canada drowning is the second leading cause of unintentional death in persons between 1 and 45.

The victim of near drowning loses the ability to stay above water. As the victim submerges, the need to breathe becomes uncontrollable. Each gasp for air draws water into the throat and causes laryngeal spasm, coughing, and choking. The victim becomes fatigued, lack of oxygen causes unconsciousness, and the victim eventually drowns. Your actions may prevent this outcome, so play it

Stop

And

First

Evaluate

Stop and quickly assess the situation. Look for items to extend your reach, such as branches, poles, or pipes. If the patient is out of reach but still conscious, throw a floatable object, preferably with a line attached. If commercial life preservers are not readily at hand, improvise. Consider the top of a cooler, an IV bag wrapped with an inflated air splint, the inflated spare tire from your vehicle, an empty gallon jug. Before attempting to enter the water weigh the risks and benefits of that action.

Determining Risks and Benefits

The Victim. Wear a personal flotation device whenever you enter the water, and place additional flotation equipment between yourself and the victim. Approach from the rear, stay defensive, and always be ready to move away. The drowning person will try to grasp at anything or anyone to keep above water. Try to offer a flotation device instead of yourself for the victim to grab.

The Water. Another risk factor to consider is the water: Is it clean? polluted? chemically unsafe? Entry into polluted or chemically unsafe water may cause immediate or long-term health hazards to the rescuer. Also consider whether the victim is in calm water or swift water. Rescue attempts involving swift water are much more dangerous and possibly fatal to the rescuer. Low-head dams and rapids require specialized rescue skills and techniques. In some cases the risk is so high that no recovery effort should be attempted.

Another water-related factor is temperature. Rescuers entering cold water without watertight clothing do so at great personal risk. Experiments conducted by the U.S. Navy in arctic regions show a strong correlation between water temperature and duration of survival (Table 14.1).

Table 14.1
Water Temperature and Survival

Water temperature °F (°C)	Duration of survival
28 (−2)	Approximately 15 minutes
32 (0)	15–30 minutes
40 (5)	30–90 minutes
50 (10)	1–4 hours
60 (16)	2–24 hours
70 (21)	3–40 hours
80 (27)	indefinite

Source: Rescue Training Associates, *Action Guide for Emergency Service Personnel* (place of publication: Brady Communication Co., 1985).

The Unconscious or Submerged Person

Caution!
Immediate rescue breathing is essential to successful resuscitation and should be done in the water.

If the victim is not responding and presumed drowned, gain access to the victim by water entry or from a boat. Approach the victim at the head. If the victim is floating face down, place the palm of your hand on the back between the shoulder blades with your arm resting on the crown of the victim's head. Place the other hand on the victim's sternum. Using the arms to immobilize the head, turn the victim face up, maintaining C-spine immobilization. A back board may be floated under the victim to assist in removal from the water. Don't begin chest compressions until the patient is moved to solid ground.

Caution!
Assume that all victims of near drowning have other injuries—protect the cervical spine.

Cold-Water Near Drowning

For years medical personnel assumed that a victim submerged for more than a few minutes could not be revived without brain damage. Brain damage remains the major factor complicating resuscitation, but more recently there are reports of persons surviving in water below 21 °C (70 °F) for up to 38 minutes. Cold water reduces the need for oxygen and activates the mammalian diving reflex (whereby blood is shunted from nonessential tissues and to the vital organs), thus extending the possibility of survival. It is believed that resuscitation is possible with victims who have been submerged up to one hour. Success seems to depend on age and water temperature. The colder the water and the younger the victim, the higher the success rate.

Caution!
Do not give up on a cold-water drowning victim until the victim is rewarmed in the emergency department.

FARMING INJURIES

Farming has often been regarded as one of the most serene vocations. New-mown hay and contented cows present a nonthreatening image to those not directly involved in agriculture. Actually, farming is the most dangerous of all trades, surpassing fivefold such notoriously dangerous occupations as logging, coal mining, and even fire-fighting. Each year, approximately 2000 people die from farm-related injuries. Of the 200,000 farming injuries a year, many are disabling. These incidents represent an estimated $5 billion in direct economic costs.

Predisposing Factors

Upon close examination, it is not difficult to see why farming accidents occur.

Long Hours and Exhaustion. The average workday for American farmers begins at about 5 A.M. and ends at sundown, or later. Although innovations have made farming much more productive, much of the work still involves intense physical labor under less-than-ideal circumstances. Many farmers also have "normal" jobs to supplement their farm income, and resume their farming activities as soon as they get off from work. Long hours and hard labor combine to create a condition all too familiar to emergency service workers—fatigue. As with the emergency services (or any other trade), fatigued workers are much more likely to be injured on the job.

Working Alone in a Remote Location. Most farming is done in areas that are inaccessible or remote by urban EMS standards. Though many farms have on-site access roads and trails, these are usually usable only by tractor or four-wheel-drive vehicles. The emphasis on a working farm is towards utilization of available land, wherever located.

Compounding the problem of remote location is the fact that the farmer or hired hand often works alone. This results in delayed recognition of injury. If the worker is injured or trapped, who will report the accident and summon help? All too often several hours pass before a farm accident is detected.

Stress. It is difficult to imagine the multiple sources of stress weighing on the average farmer. The farmer must function as an agronomist, parent, veterinarian, mechanic, and accountant. Fatigue is an obvious source of physical stress, but mental stress may actually be greater.

Agricultural Injuries

Combine these predisposing factors with animals, machinery, chemicals, and other farm hazards and you have an environment where trauma is likely. Common injuries include chemical and thermal burns, suffocation, asphyxiation, hazardous material exposure, and multi-system trauma, including crush injury. As with any trauma, time is a determinant of outcome in farm injuries. Since many of these injuries are not even detected for hours, the EMT may find that the "golden hour" has passed some time prior to arrival at the scene.

Barring complicating factors such as entrapment and a lack of access, EMTs should initiate rapid evaluation of the patient's condition, paying attention to the ABCs. Package the patient (see Chapter 13) and transport. Advanced life support (ALS) can often make a critical difference in patient survival, and an ALS unit should be dispatched simultaneously with basic life support (BLS) units.

While advanced life support is desirable, rural responders should not delay transport to await a distant ALS provider. Perform basic life support and initiate transport as quickly as possible! If necessary, paramedics, and physicians can be met somewhere en route to hospital.

Caution!
Responders to rural trauma incidents should be aware of the availability and capability of air medical support in their response areas.

Helicopters are valuable assets in rural trauma operations. Rapid transfer of victims, deployment of rural ALS, and transport of medical/rescue specialists and equipment are but a few of the services helicopter units provide. Since capabilities vary from service to service, pre-incident in-service training is recommended.

The diversity of potential injury is as great as the number of current farming operations. EMS providers should actively seek to obtain orientation to agricultural activities common to their area, and adapt plans to treatment protocol.

Caution!
There are serious dangers to rescuers not adequately trained in farm rescue techniques. Usual extrication techniques may more seriously injure patient and rescuer.

MINE RESCUE

There are three primary types of mining operations in North America.

Quarrying (Open Pit)

This type of mining is used primarily to remove slabs of marble, granite, or limestone. This is accomplished by drilling and splitting the rock. Large slabs of rock are lifted by crane and transported for final cutting. A similar operation is used to make gravel or stone. The stone is drilled and then blasted into manageable size. These rocks are processed through a crusher to yield a salable product.

Strip Mining

This type of mine involves removing the entire top of a mountain or other surface to reach the minerals beneath. State and federal regulations limit the surface area to be mined, and most states require the area to be returned to its original elevation.

If either of these types of mines is in your area, a site visit is recommended. There are a few things to look for and consider during the visit. Learn the access roads and the location of the mine office. The mine office is the most likely staging area in an emergency. Depending on the situation, your job may be no more than to wait at the office for the patient to be brought out. Rarely are the roads in and out of a mine designed for ambulances; in most cases, other means of transportation will be required. Gaining access to the injured patient may take an extended period, so be sure to take all the equipment needed. Obtain orders for patient treatment before entering the mine, which may be very deep and block radio transmissions. Also, radio traffic may be restricted if explosives are nearby. Injuries associated with quarry and strip mining are primarily amputations, crush injuries, and falls. Not as common but often as fatal is drowning when excavation breaks into underground water sources.

Deep Mining (Shaft Mining)

This type of mining uses the ground, which may be several hundred feet deep. Elevators move up and down the main shaft, and air is pumped in and water is pumped out through adjacent vertical shafts. Horizontal passageways extend from the vertical shaft at different levels and directions, and each has many smaller tunnels (Figure 14.1). Although the size and heights of these tunnels depend on the size of the mineral vein, a height of 3 or 4 feet is typical. This type of mining is the most dangerous because miners are constantly exposed to structural collapses, methane explosions, oxygen deficiency, electrical hazards, and compressed air. Total darkness, dust, and heavy machinery are constant risks.

Because of the high hazard potential and the inability of local EMS coordinators to cope with the hazards in mine rescue, commercial mines usually have a special rescue team. These team members are familiar with the mine layout, danger signs, shoring techniques, debris removal, and emergency medicine. When responding to an emergency at a large mine, report to the mine office and follow instructions. You will probably not have to enter the mine, but you will need to be prepared for accident victims brought to the surface.

At an independent (bootleg) mine, the work force and support staff are usually less. Report to the lift operator and determine the scope of the problem. Miners from other mines will usually respond. If no one with knowledge about the mine can be found, call the local mine safety office for advice and assistance. Stand by for qualified mine rescuers and assist as required. As a general rule, never enter a mine without at least three experienced miners.

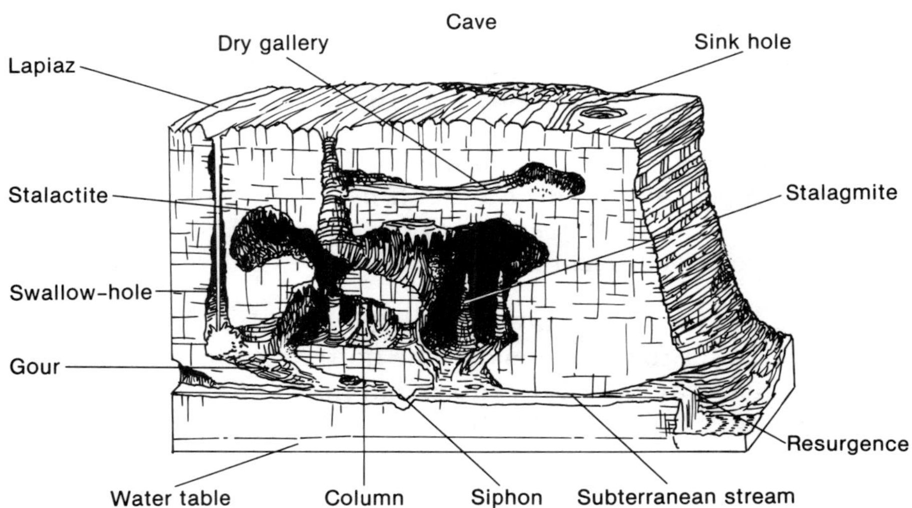

FIGURE 14.1 Deep mine with vertical and horizontal shafts.

CAVE RESCUE

Although EMTs and fire-fighters are often called for someone lost or injured in a cave, they are probably the least prepared for this uniquely hostile environment. For example, bunker coats are too bulky to fit through small passages, fire-fighter's boots provide unsafe footing, and some emergency medical equipment, such as a Stokes basket, is too big to negotiate narrow, twisting passageways. Standard drug boxes and medical packs are poorly suited to the underground environment, and lights need to be able to sustain 8 to 10 hours of continuous usage.

Agencies with caves in their area should contact the National Speleological Society to obtain the name of the nearest grotto, or chapter. Members can provide information on local caves and extend assistance. In an emergency, the EMT may also call Scott Air Force Base (800-851-3051) and request the Cave Rescue Coordinator. Coordination centers for state civil defense have listings of qualified cave rescue personnel in each area.

Types of Caves

Solution Caves. These caves are the most commonly encountered. Passageways may be vertical or horizontal and are of two basic types. Phreatic passages tend to be large and smooth-walled with mostly dry, level floors. Vadosa passages are formed by fast-moving water and tend to be irregular in shape with narrow, fluted passages that may contain active waterways.

Talus Caves. These are formed by fallen rock between ridges at the base of a mountain. Although not really caves, people do get hurt in them. The irregularity of passageways and their instability are added hazards.

Lava Tubes. These are formed in molten lava when the outside cools faster than the inside. The hotter lava inside flows out of the center, leaving hollow tubes that may extend several hundred feet and intersect with other tubes. These caves also tend to be unstable.

Cave Problems

There are several basic problems that must be overcome if the patient and the rescuer are to come out of the cave alive. Keep in mind that patient transport is often difficult; it may take hours to move the patient a mere 100 feet. Rescue may take as little as 1 to 2 hours, or it may take days. Be prepared to coordinate a large number of persons for an extended period.

Darkness. The darkness in a cave is absolute, and rescuers must carry three sources of light with them. Each person should have a helmet-mounted light capable of 8 to 10 hours of continuous operation. Spare bulbs and batteries should be carried in a pack. A waterproof flashlight with extra batteries and bulbs should be included as a second source of illumination. The third source of light may be a supply of candles with matches. These are used when repair of a main light is needed or when waiting, and the EMT can expect a lot of waiting. Carbon lights are popular for exploration, but should not be used around the patient during rescue, as the open flames may injure the patient and/or equipment.

Water. Most caves, especially those formed by water, are natural drains for the world above. Water temperature in American caves averages 55 °F. Immersion in water of this temperature will cause hypothermia within a few minutes.

Many caves flood with rainwater. Therefore, trends in weather must be monitored prior to entering a cave. Every year persons are trapped inside caves by flooding. In some locations this happens so frequently that cavers stock food, water, and dry clothing inside caves to wait out the flood. Only cave divers should be used to rescue trapped cavers. The National Cave Rescue Commission (NCRC) has available trained cave divers.

Passageways. Passageways in caves tend to be very irregular and vary from very large to very tight. Rescuers may have to compress their chest to get through the small passageways. They may feel claustrophobic even if they have never experienced this feeling before. Some passageways are so small and have so many turns and twists that the victim has no choice but to stay underground until the injury heals enough for self-rescue. An alternative in such cases is the mine rescue drill, which drills a 24-inch shaft to the victim's position. This is tedious work, for it takes a whole day to drill through 50 feet of limestone. Moreover, to get the drill in position may take several days; caves are seldom near roads and the drill has to be positioned almost directly over the victim.

Air Temperature and Air Movement. The cave temperature generally corresponds to the area's annual temperature, and is approximately 52 to 60 °F in most caves in the U.S. Temperature is the greatest environmental hazard. The patient and the rescuer lose heat in four ways. Awareness of causes of heat loss and preventative measures will increase both the patient's and the EMT's chance of survival:

- Conduction: heat loss by body contact with rocks, water, and mud.
- Radiation: direct loss of heat, especially if clothing is inadequate.
- Convection: heat loss by air currents moving over the body.
- Respiration: loss of heat through breathing.

An uninjured person can keep warm by moving around and by eating high-carbohydrate foods. An entrapped cave victim will not have this option, so the EMT must protect the individual from the environment. Provide blankets and dry clothing, and protect the victim from water.

Air Inside Caves. With very few exceptions caves, unlike mines, tend to ventilate themselves well with changes in barometric pressure. Therefore, the rescuer seldom needs to ventilate or wear breathing apparatus. Support operations on the surface should use extreme care when setting up portable generators or vehicles to avoid introducing lethal fumes into the cave. Carbon dioxide and carbon monoxide will pool lower in the cave and may displace oxygen.

Route Finding. It is unlikely that the EMT will have access to a map of the cave, or familiarity with a cave-map and the cave. Most caves have one or two entrances, multiple main passageways, and many side passages. Upon entering, make mental notes of the route; look back often to picture the exit route. Consider marking your path with removable markers. Caves commonly have a maze where several tunnels converge, and it is very easy to get lost or disoriented.

Equipment. Most equipment on ambulances is either useless or improperly packaged for cave rescue. Stoke baskets are too large to negotiate narrow passageways. Scoop stretchers have proven unsafe underground. The best stretcher for underground rescue is a modified Neills-Robertson with an added support frame.

Drag sheets, made from conveyor belting, are useful for pulling people through small passages. The skid litter works well but is easily damaged by abrasion from rocks and mud.

Rescue Assistance and Training. When there is need for a cave rescue, contact the National Cave Rescue Commission (NCRC) through Scott Air Force Base. The NCRC maintains a rescue call list of teams throughout the United States. They can provide advisers, cae teams, and cave divers. The NCRC also conducts training classes. For information, write to the National Cave Rescue Commission, Cave Avenue, Huntsville, Alabama 35810.

MASS CASUALTIES

The most important aspect of handling a mass casualty incident is preparation—there is absolutely no substitute. Some maintain that preparing for mass casualty incidents is a waste of time since they occur so rarely. They are indeed rare, but preparation for them is far from a waste of time. A flexible mass casualty plan will be useful far beyond the disaster situation for which it was intended. A flexible plan is one that establishes protocol starting on a small scale and increasing to the disaster itself with a scope wide enough to include special nonmedical disaster situtations.

Knowledge gained from mass casualty training can be applied daily. In a sense, anytime the number of victims exceeds the number of medical personnel, a mass casualty incident has occurred. Even in a situation of only two or three patients to one rescuer, the principles of handling mass casualties apply. Scene evaluation, request for additional resources, and triage are used just as in large disasters involving dozens of patients. Beyond medical emergencies, the disaster plan is useful in many other situations, such as natural disasters and exposure to hazardous materials.

Preparing for mass casualty incidents also makes communities aware of resources. It exposes weaknesses in the system so that components in the emergency network can be improved. Various agencies learn to work together and share expertise.

Organization

Key members of a community's emergency agencies should meet and set up a disaster committee. This committee should include individuals from all agencies responsible for emergency services, as well as local government and medical representatives. They should develop a disaster plan that delegates duties and responsibilities to the various agencies. The plan should be flexible so that it can be changed as the program progresses. The plans of other communities should be reviewed for guidance.

Another early step is to recognize what resources are presently available to the community for handing disasters. In taking this inventory, keep in mind probable causes of mass casualty incidents. The presence of airports, harbors, factories, and mines increases the potential for mass injury incidents. These should receive attention, but the possible sources of more unlikely disasters should also be addressed. Agency personnel should compile a list of equipment and resources needed for all of these disasters.

Publications, government agencies, and comparable towns or cities should be consulted. Once needs are determined, resources should be examined to see if local needs can be met. Records of items, access, and availability should be noted for the community disaster resource manual. Many businesses are willing to provide equipment on an emergency basis that may be used for years (consider construction firms, rental agencies, and building supply companies). Schools, churches, and factories may provide shelter. Strategic dispersal of equipment such as cots, blankets, and food may be worthwhile. National agencies such as the Federal Emergency Management Agency (FEMA) and the American Red Cross may provide assistance.

There are alternatives for meeting needs not locally available. Mutual aid agreements with nearby towns can be established. Also consider nearby military and other government facilities that may possess needed resources. Local state or federal agencies have access to federal and state surplus warehouses, where equipment may be purchased at greatly reduced prices. In some cases state or federal grants may also be available.

As equipment needs are defined, the disaster committee should compile a manual that includes material and technical assistance resources. It is vital to include information about how to quickly obtain their resources and get them to the scene. Hospital field teams should be established (if available) and trained in field techniques and equipment. A chain of command should be established for notification within each level, defining who is responsible for specific tasks in the disaster plan.

> **Caution!**
> Who is in charge? Address this issue in your plan to avoid conflict during a disaster.

There are many opinions regarding who is in charge. These may give rise to emotional and legal arguments. State, federal, and local laws vary. By having a plan, participants can agree upon areas of responsibility and work together for the good of the community.

Once the disaster plan is established, it must be practiced. Small, specialized drills that allow experience and expertise to accumulate should be conducted first. Copies of the disaster plan should be distributed to appropriate agencies; there a working knowledge of the plan should be developed, especially by those in leadership positions.

Principles of Disaster Management

Approach from upwind if there is any chance of fire or hazardous materials. Park the rescue vehicle where it is accessible but out of the way.

Initial Report. A good initial size-up and report may take time away from treating patients, but will probably save lives in the long run by insuring immediate provision of much-needed assistance. Include estimated number of patients in the critical, serious, and minor categories, the best route of approach, the location of staging and command areas, and any special resources needed. If indicated, request that the disaster plan be implemented. This would establish the necessary communications for activating mutual aid, medical field team response, and other aspects of the disaster plan.

Setting Up Command. One of the biggest weaknesses of many disaster responses is the failure to establish command. This invariably leads to mass confusion, duplication, or omission. Identification of command is simply indispensable for an effective disaster response.

Generally, the first person at the scene is in command until others arrive. Therefore, the initial command point will be the scene vehicle. This should be announced so that arriving units report to the command location for specific assignments rather than immediately proceeding with unorganized activities that lead to duplication or omission. The initial command center may be changed once leadership personnel from other agencies arrive and determine the needs for the incident. The command center should be in a location where a good overview of the incident is possible. The command should be well marked and crews should report to this location. Within the command center should be a representative from each agency with radio capability to that agency. This will cut down on disorganized, duplicate, and conflicting transmissions and prevent individuals on the scene from overwhelming the local dispatch center. As soon as possible, on-scene radio frequencies should be designated.

Caution!
All communications at the scene should go through the command center for relay to the dispatch center.

Staging Area. As vehicles and personnel arrive, it is desirable to locate them appropriately. One or more persons should be assigned to direct incoming units to a staging area and call for them as directed by the command center. Be sure vehicles are positioned to permit leaving or moving as needed. Many incidents tie up emergency vehicles, preventing movement as needed for rescue, fire, or patient transport. The staging area should allow ambulances to locate adjacent to the triage area for rapid patient loading and removal. It may be necessary to have a separate staging area for ambulances.

It takes discipline to keep unneeded personnel away from the action, but in some cases too many people in a very limited area detracts from the response. The command center should indicate where specific personnel are needed and direct others to the staging area to be summoned as the need arises. This allows better awareness and control of personnel.

Triage. Triage—sorting patients and treating them in order of medical priority—is one of the most important components of disaster management.

> **Caution!**
> The principle of disaster management is to do the greatest good for the greatest number. Without an organized system of treating patients, inappropriate and untimely care will surely result.

Triage establishes patient categories so that the most seriously injured patients (except those with little or no chance for survival) are treated first. It is inappropriate for patients with either minor injuries or with a poor prognosis (cardiac arrest or severe head injuries, severe burns) to reduce the ability of rescuers to manage those patients with severe bleeding or other conditions with a greater chance of survival. Triage is divided into four categories:

- Critical: needs immediate care; in danger of dying
- Serious: needs care soon but not in immediate life-threatening danger
- Minor: ambulatory or nonurgent
- Dead or dying: little or no chance of survival, even with immediate care

  (Note: Some jurisdictions utilize numeric and/or color coding to identify categories.)

It is important that the disaster plan recognize these categories and have an easy method of identifying them. Color coded triage tags are available while colored flagging tape may provide a less expensive alternative.

The triage area should be close to both the incident site and the transport vehicle staging area. In the mass casualty setting, immediate transport of victims is seldom indicated since personnel are needed to stay on the scene and render lifesaving care. Initial triage takes place where the victims are found. In order of medical priority, the victims are taken to the triage area where they are reassessed, receive limited emergency care, and are delegated for transport in order of medical priority. The triage area should be upwind if any hazardous materials exist, and should be well marked. Color-coded cones, tarps, or flags can be used to identify the different sections for the different patient categories. The section for the critically and seriously injured patients should be most accessible to medical equipment and transport vehicles. Patients with minor injuries may be located nearby, but out of the way. These patients, though categorized as having minor injuries, should be watched by someone for any sign of deterioration that would indicate upgrading their medical priority. A triage officer who is familiar with disaster management should coordinate the triage area. The triage officer directs where incoming patients are placed, reassesses their condition, and changes it if indicated. The triage officer also directs patient care within the triage area, and coordinates outgoing patient flow with the transport officer.

Noncommand Officers

Transport Officer. This person must be aware of hospital resources (number of beds, specific medical capabilities) and directs patients to the most appropriate facility.

Landing Zone (LZ) Officer. This person is in charge of setting up a safe and appropriate landing area for helicopters. It should be of adequate size and without surrounding obstructions. It should be near the triage area, but not where helicopter approach or landing will cause excessive rotor blast and noise. This officer is also in charge of communications with the aircraft and general safety within the LZ area.

Communications Officer. This individual designates radio frequencies and coordinates interagency communications, both on the scene and with the dispatch center.

Rescue Officer. This individual is in charge of rescue operations at the scene.

Fire Officer. This officer has charge of fire or hazardous materials on the scene.

Collectively, these officers coordinate with those serving in the command area. They relay requests for additional resources through the command center and coordinate activities at the incident site. Other personnel may eventually be needed as well: chaplains, support personnel for food and drink, lighting and shelter. Once the survivors are cared for, the dead must be dealt with. In some cases, they cannot be moved until after a preliminary investigation. Body bags and temporary morgues may be required.

Drills

Once the basic principles of disaster management have been acquired, practical drills should be held. Drills start out on a small scale and increase in scope and difficulty as crews become more skilled. Drills allow a gradual building of knowledge and abilities.

Tabletop Drills. Agencies can practice "tabletop" drills—those where incidents are represented in print. These are easy to set up and conduct, and provide invaluable experience. Personnel discuss appropriate courses of action for disaster management by the various responding groups. These do much to review disaster management and available resources, and coordinate alternate actions.

Communication Drills. Agencies may simulate an incident for the communication portion of the disaster plan. All notifications are carried out, resources are confirmed, hospitals alerted and bed availability ensured. Communication drills serve to update information, confirm telephone numbers, and define availability of various resources.

Small Field Walk-through Exercises. A mass casualty situation is described and personnel from various agencies describe their response, including how they would approach, where staging and triage areas would be established, and what additional resources would be needed. A critique should immediately follow all practice and real exercises.

Small-scale Drills. These may use either individual or multiple agencies. A small-scale drill should consist of enough patients to require principles of disaster management, but not so many as to overwhelm participants. Principles of proper approach, initial reports, and setting up a command center and staging and triage areas should be stressed. As personnel increase their disaster management skills the drills can be made larger by adding other agencies and complications. It may also be valuable to initiate some surprise drills at this point.

Large-scale Drills. Opinions differ over whether these should be announced or unannounced. It is usually very difficult to keep large-scale drills a secret. At least the first few should probably be announced. It is imperative that they be well planned. The time and place should be such that it does not unnecessarily interfere with the rest of the community. It should not compromise the ability of the participating agencies to respond to the actual community needs that might occur during the drill. The community should be forewarned to avoid unnecessary alarm or panic. This also serves the purpose of having bystanders at the scene and adds realism to the drill. The comfort of the victims should also be considered. Extremes of heat or cold should be avoided. Makeup of victims (moulage) or use of injury description cards adds reality to the drill. It is very important that observers be present at the communications center (recordings should be made of all communications and times noted) and the disaster site (including the command post, staging area, triage area, and transportation area). Observers should be selected to watch for skills in which they have unique expertise: rescue, hazardous materials, and patient care. Participating hospitals should also have observers.

> **Caution!**
> Units should not run emergency traffic, and unnecessary hazards should not be simulated.

It is impractical for crews to carry out patient care with equipment that might be needed on a real call at any time. Organizers should establish ground rules concerning what should be carried out and what should be simulated. Many drills simply have crews write on the patient's card what treatment they would render. Any gear actually used is recovered immediately before leaving the hospital.

Critique

It is essential to hold a critique after each practice and real incident. Representatives from participating agencies and appointed observers should report on what was done well or what needed improvement. Opportunity for questions and discussion should be allowed. Once the overall critique is held, individual agencies should hold their own review. Once the disaster committee considers the agencies prepared, a surprise drill may be appropriate.

> **Caution!**
> A disaster plan must be flexible yet structured so that it can be implemented on a graduated basis that allows its use in small-scale disasters as well as major ones.

AIRCRAFT CRASHES

Aircraft accidents pose unusual problems in rescue/extrication, fire and other hazards, and scene protection. Rescuers must be aware of these to facilitate a quick and effective operation that does not compromise safety or the postcrash investigation. While training programs exist for airport-based crash-fire-rescue teams, few have been directed to emergency personnel in the community who have less exposure and specialized equipment to deal with aircraft emergencies.

The information presented here applies mainly to general aviation aircraft (civilian-owned) in an off-airport crash setting. This material is a brief overview and should not be interpreted as a complete instruction resource. You are encouraged to seek further information and instruction from other resources.

General Considerations

Most nonairport emergency personnel have limited knowledge of aircraft and their components. Therefore, the folowing information is provided.

Emergency Locator Transmitter (ELT). This is a device required on most aircraft that transmits an emergency signal on frequency 121.50 MHz. This device can be triggered manually or by impact. Some have two-way communications capability if the aircraft's radios still function. This is significant since many scanners and programmable radios used in EMS are capable of picking up these emergency frequencies. The ELT signal has a distinctive warbling sound.

Aircraft Engines. Some aircraft have piston or reciprocal engines; others use jet or jet-prop engines. Like any engine, each poses potential hazards. Rescuers should use caution around propeller-driven aircraft since movement of the prop could restart the engine. Hot exhaust stacks and jet blast/intakes pose safety and/or fire dangers.

Aircraft Structural Components and Related Hazards. Because aircraft must be lightweight, construction consists of many strong but lightweight materials. Some may require special fire suppression agents and techniques (for example, magnesium alloys burn violently and resist extinguishment with water). Steel or stainless steel parts spark and create fire potential. Other aircraft components, such as titanium or graphite composites, may be especially resistant to normal extrication procedures because of their strength and flexibility.

Fuel and Fuel System. In highway crashes emergency personnel must deal with two common types of fuel: gasoline and diesel fuel. Essentially, the same can be said for aircraft accidents. The two major types of aircraft fuel are gasoline (AVGAS) and kerosene (JET–A, which is similar to diesel). The type of fuel can be determined by the type of engine (AVGAS in piston engines, JET–A in jet or jet-prop engines), visual inspection, or each fuel's distinctive odor. In any crash the presence of a fuel leak creates added hazards. Precautions for leaking aircraft fuel are fairly standard, but control methods require knowledge of the craft and its fuel system. For instance, fuel valve switches, fire suppression handles, and the fuel pump may be utilized to control leaking fuel. Rubber or wooden plugs may be used to control some leaks while crimping may slow those from exposed fuel lines.

Fuel Cells or Tanks. The location, size, and construction of fuel tanks vary by aircraft type. Most smaller fixed-wing aircraft have fuel tanks in each of the wings. Some aircraft may have fuel tanks in wing tip tanks, and auxiliary tanks mounted inside the cabin under the cabin floor (common in helicopters) or in external-mounted pods (military aircraft). Some of these tanks are designed to resist rupture and to seal off leaks.

Electrical Systems. It is important for fire/rescue personnel to disable the craft's electrical system to reduce fire hazards. This can be done by either disconnecting the battery(s) or placing the cockpit battery or master switch in the off position. If possible, both of these procedures should be done. In many small aircraft the master switch is often a red rocker switch on the control panel near the ignition and will be labeled *master*. The number of batteries and their location will vary on different aircraft. In most newer single-engine aircraft it will be in the nose area near the fire wall; twin-engine planes may have the battery either in the nose or tail compartments. Airplane batteries look much like a car battery and many have a single quick-disconnect knob on the front, which works with a single counterclockwise turn.

Hydraulic System. Hydraulic systems are used on larger aircraft and many rotary-wing aircraft to assist with the operation of various aircraft controls and systems (flaps, landing gear, control surfaces), much like the power steering system in cars. Cutting into any lines of an intact hydraulic system may cause this hot fluid to be released under pressure in a fine mist, which is highly flammable as well as irritating to the skin and eyes. A good rule of thumb is to avoid cutting through any aircraft lines during rescue operations.

Caution!
Burning hydraulic fluid produces toxic vapors—*use full protective gear!*

Aircraft Oxygen. Many aircraft have oxygen tanks on board. Some of these will be standard tanks while many military, and a growing number of EMS aircraft, have liquid oxygen (LOX) systems. Emergency personnel should treat damaged oxygen tanks with appropriate caution.

Incident Reporting

An air traffic controller (ATC) is a Federal Aviation Agency (FAA) employee found at larger airports who coordinates aircraft traffic. The ATC will notify the proper authorities of an air accident. If an aircraft is on a flight plan or has declared an emergency the ATC may be able to provide valuable information: type of aircraft, tail number, number of occupants and fuel load.

The tail number (also known as the *N* number because civilian non-experimental planes registered in the U.S. have a registration starting with the letter N) is required to be displayed and usually appears as large figures on the side of the fuselage in the tail area. It is important to ascertain an accurate and complete registration number of the accident craft and report it to the flight service station (FSS) as soon as possible. Damage or fire may make this number illegible. Disturbing the wreckage should be avoided. A small tag showing the N number may also be found on the control panel of many planes.

The FAA has overall responsibility for investigation of aircraft accidents. The FSS is responsible for local search and rescue operations. Other agencies involved include the National Transportation Safety Board (NTSB), which makes recommendations to the FAA and Civil Air Patrol (CAP), a branch of the U.S. Air Force that assists in search operations for missing aircraft. When there is an aircraft in trouble, but actual crash (or location of impact) is unknown, certain information should be obtained: the location and time that witnesses observed the aircraft, the general direction of travel and altitude, and a general description (size, type and number of engines, color and markings, etc.). The weather at the time, fire, smoke, or parts coming from the plane, unusual sounds or maneuvers are potentially important. Also determine if an impact was seen or heard and if smoke was seen from the suspected impact area. A description of the terrain in the area is also important.

Whether a crash is confirmed or only reported, local emergency services need only call one of the FAA-operated flight facilities serving the area to activate all needed assistance. If in doubt, look under the *U.S. Government* listing in the local phone book under the subheading of transportation. Assistance may come from several facilities: Flight Service Station, Flight Standards District Office (FSDO), General Aviation District Office (GADO), Pilot Weather Briefing Service.

Search Operations

When the local Flight Service Station (FSS) is notified of a missing aircraft it will coordinate search operations. Initial efforts include attempts to establish radio contact, checking for ELT or other distress signals, checking airport parking areas for the missing craft, and monitoring any reports of aircraft in trouble. If the aircraft is not located during this phase of the search, a full-scale operation by air and ground teams is initiated.

Air and ground search teams are coordinated to cover the areas of highest probability. The possibility area is roughly a circle with its center at the last known position of the aircraft and its radius being the maximum distance that could be traveled in any direction until fuel exhaustion would occur. Within this circle is an area of probability based on projected flight path, radar or radio contacts, witness reports and weather conditions. As the probable areas are covered the search area is expanded to cover other areas of the circle.

If a crash is confirmed, it should be reported to the FSS (or its equivalent) immediately upon confirmation by emergency or other qualified personnel. Information previously discussed should be provided to the extent known (Table 14.2). The flight service station (or an equivalent) should take care of all necessary aviation accident notifications.

TABLE 14.2
Essential Crash Information

Aircraft:	Number of aircraft, description (markings, size, type, military/civilian, tail number)
Location:	Access to nearest town, major roadway, airport
Victims:	Aircraft victims, ground casualities and general condition
Special Needs:	Rescue, hazardous materials, military, fire
Other:	Call-back number, contact person, and location to meet arriving teams

Response

Approach and Positioning (General Guidelines—Fire or No Fire). Often access to the crash site may be limited by terrain, vegetation, or ground conditions. As personnel and vehicles arrive, position support operations upwind and uphill from the crash for better protection from heat, smoke, or leaking fuel. Drivers must be especially alert to avoid hitting victims thrown from the wreckage—especially where smoke, vegetation, poor lighting, or weather reduce visibility. The same care should be used to avoid hitting pieces of wreckage, since the vehicle could be disabled and valuable evidence or property destroyed. Vehicle parking should ensure that units will not be blocked by one another and can be quickly repositioned should the need arise. Fire suppression units should be positioned closest to the wreckage without other vehicles in between. Crews should set up to provide maximum protection for occupied areas of the wreckage—especially exits.

Personnel and vehicles should also avoid common danger areas in plane crashes including engine danger areas (intake, exhaust, and propellers), under wings or other wreckage subject to collapse, near wheels, fuel tanks, or other components that may explode from heat exposure. Gullies, ditches, and other areas where spilled fuel may collect or areas in line with weapons (in front or behind) should also be avoided. Rescue crews should practice caution and safety as the situation demands.

Scene Considerations

An initial report should be given within a few moments of the first arriving unit after a quick survey is made to determine need for additional resources, hazards, number of casualties, and aircraft information. This data should be relayed to other incoming units as well as the FSS. While care of victims, extrication, and control of hazards takes priority, the scene should be preserved to the extent possible. The crash scene should be treated just like a crime scene in order to assure the most accurate investigation possible. If any bodies or pieces of wreckage have to be moved, try to record their location with photography, ID tags, or survey flags. Note if victims have restraint belts on and any evidence of belt failure. Any alteration of aircraft controls or switches should be documented. Deceased victims should be left in place until the NTSB authorities arrive. Try to document temporary evidence such as ice and snow.

Fire Safety and Suppression in Aircraft Accidents

Even when no fire is initially present crews should work under the assumption that there is an extreme and continuous danger of fire.

All personnel should use full protective gear and nonessential persons and vehicles should remain in a staging area. Shut down vehicles not in use. Apply and maintain a blanket of foam on fuel spills, hot engine components, and any other potential ignition source. If foam is not available water may be used sparingly, since water has no blanketing properties and will spread the fuel hazard. Added hose lines, as they become available, should be strategically positioned peripherally to protect rescuers should fire break out. Measures should be implemented to control fuel leaks by diking or trenches, and potential ignition sources should be eliminated. Fire prevention takes on added significance when access to the crash site by adequate fire suppression equipment is not possible.

Aircraft Accidents with Fire. The classic characteristic of aircraft fires are that they reach an extreme intensity in a very short period. When an aircraft fuselage is engulfed in fire it takes 90 to 120 seconds to burn through the metal skin. If evacuation does not take place within this time occupants usually die from burns, exposure to smoke, or lack of oxygen. Initial fire response in some communities may be limited by personnel and equipment. While this response might be overwhelmed by the crash of a large aircraft, smaller general aviation airplanes contain less fuel and fires can be more easily managed. It is also possible that the crash will not be accessible to fire fighting equipment. In such cases the fire will have probably consumed the aircraft by the time rescuers arrive.

Caution!
Controlling the fire to allow rescue is more important than actual extinguishment.

While foam is the agent of choice in aircraft fires, an initial quick attack with water lines using fog patterns should be conducted unless foam lines are set up and ready for immediate use. Then, if needed, foam or larger diameter lines can be set up. As in other fires, approach should be made from upwind. The first goal is to open and maintain rescue pathways. The primary discharge of the agent should be made along the line of the fuselage at an angle to push the fire/smoke/heat away from the occupied area of the craft—especially at the exits. The key is to keep the occupied portions of wreckage cool enough for survival while protecting rescuers and maintaining an escape route. The largest most survivable section of wreckage should take highest fire-fighting priority. If the fire is in a wing or engine area away from the fuselage a heat shield action with a fog or water curtain should be used. Emphasis must be placed on the value of a foam blanket, full protective gear, and backup lines placed to cover personnel inside the immediate fire area.

Caution!
There is constant threat of reignition (flashback) when fighting a fire where amounts of fuel are involved.

Wheel fires should be approached from fore or aft direction to the wheel and never from in line with the axle since a burning or overheated wheel may explode and fragments are more likely to project in that direction. Magnesium components often found in aircraft wheels will require special fire suppression measures. Small compartment fires may be handled with extinguishers. Aircraft inspection and maintenance doors often provide good access for application of fire agents in enclosed compartment areas.

Caution!
Magnesium fire + water = explosion. Do not use water on magnesium fires!

Aircraft Rescue

As in any rescue, first priority should be given to overviewing the scene for the best approach, hazards, and special needs. Fire safety, hazard control, and wreckage stabilization should be performed as needed. Beware of parts of the aircraft subject to collapse. Determine the location of all victims within the craft and make extrication plans accordingly. Use of equipment and personnel staging areas will help avoid confusion. As in vehicle rescue, doors and windows are the preferred means of gaining access.

Doors. If normal means of access/exit are not possible, aircraft have a wide variety of escape/evacution systems. Opening methods vary among aircraft and types of doors, hatches, or canopies, but instructions are usually printed on the outside of the craft at the release or handle. If forcible entry is required, use of standard extrication tools will usually be effective. Latching mechanisms may vary in location and number. Many doors will have latches at the top and bottom. Smaller aircraft may have exposed door hinges allowing door removal with nothing more than a phillips screwdriver.

Windows. The second choice for extrication is the windows. Look for emergency escape windows, since other windows may prove too small to allow victim removal. As with doors, exit windows will usually have visible opening instructions and opening mechanisms in and outside the aircraft. Many are simply mounted in a rubber molding and can be pushed out at the corners with little effort. Window exits on larger craft usually open to the inside.

Nonexit windows may be small and difficult to remove. They are usually plexiglass and may be removed by cutting a small hole at one corner, grasping the rubber molding surrounding the window, and pulling it free. The windscreen or windshield usually consists of layers of laminated glass. This can be cut with an axe or other tools, but the victim must be protected from flying glass and sharp edges.

Some aircraft have cut-through areas marked on the fuselage: The words *cut here* with a yellow or black border area indicate the cut pattern. These cut areas are usually found on military aircraft, but may be present on some civilian crafts as well.

The last and most complicated method of access is cutting through the aircraft body. As in cars, the structural makeup of the craft will make cutting through the body difficult and time consuming. Because aircraft structures are often made with extremely hard metals, common rescue tools (saws-all, air chisel) may not be effective. If using this last resort, the rescuer must locate an area between structural members and avoid various lines that will undermine and quite possibly defeat your efforts. As in a car, the top or roof of the aircraft will usually have fewer obstructions than the bottom. If it is a high wing aircraft, access through the roof should be well clear of the wing area. Once inside, tripping the seat release or seat-back lever (if so equipped) may gain needed room. Also, most aircraft seats fit into a track and can be removed by unbolting them. There are several types of restraint belt systems found on aircraft and rescuers should be familiar with them all. They are easily released with a single motion, but should be cut if normal release is not immediately achieved.

Rescue Equipment. Most rescue tools used in vehicle extrication are also effective in aircraft accidents. Because air crashes often have poor access and create confined working spaces, small lightweight equipment is often preferred over heavy and/or bulky equipment. Tools which have limited friction or sparking potential are preferred. The selection of extrication devices will be greatly affected by crash access, fire and stabilization hazards, type of aircraft and the circumstances of the entrapment. The following are some items that may be expecially useful in the aircraft setting:

- Wooden or rubber plugs for fuel line leaks
- Felt or rubber pads to cover sharp or jagged edges
- Harness-cutting knife for seat belts
- Serrated fire axe
- Metal-cutting hatchet and tin snips
- Cable cutter (most standard wire cutters will not work on aircraft control cables)
- Assortment of non-sparking hand tools
- Porta-powers with wedge and ram accessories

While rescuers should utilize protective gear, efforts should also be made to protect victims during extrication. Finally, it should never be assumed all victims have been rescued until a search of the wreckage and surrounding area has been completed. Don't overlook the possibility of victims other than those on the aircraft.

Casualties. Injuries and their treatment are similar to those found in car crashes—they may range from minor to severe. Emergency medical personnel should keep in mind, however, that deceleration may be much more extreme and four dimensional. These injuries are often complicated by entrapment, inaccessibility to the crash site, and exposure to the elements. The extreme forces in air accidents often produce horrifying injuries or numbers of casualties that may have psychological effects on rescuers long after the incident is over. Historically, immediate counseling has proven to be very useful in helping EMTs deal with the emotional trauma of these and other types of mishaps.

Special Rescue Situations

Military Aircraft. The appropriate military service should be notified immediately. They may provide valuable information and assistance. These aircraft are often of much stronger construction, which may deter extrication efforts. There is also the danger of explosive jettison or ejection systems and weapons. Accidental activation of the canopy jettison or pilot ejection systems pose a high potential for injury or death to both rescuers and air crews. In general, when dealing with military aircraft, avoid touching any brightly colored handle, switch, or button. Commonly, ejection and weapon-fire mechanisms will be red, red- and white-striped, or yellow- and black-striped.

Hazardous Cargo. Both civilian and military aircraft may carry a variety of other dangerous cargo. Even if placarded it may not be visible so crews should assume, as in any accident, the possibility of hazardous materials and take appropriate measures.

Crashes into Water. Special dive rescue assistance should be be summoned immediately. Remember, fuel/oil/hydraulic slicks on the water's surface will not only create a fire hazard, but possibly injure victims and rescue personnel alike. If the aircraft is partially submerged efforts should be made to secure it from sinking or drifting. Added flotation and anchor lines should be attached. A marker buoy should be attached to assist in locating the plane, should it sink. Never cut into the body of a floating aircraft since to do so might allow the air bubble within to escape and cause the wreckage to sink before rescue can be accomplished. In general, entry should be below water level.

Pulling the wreckage from the water to effect rescue should only be considered as a last resort since doing so may displace a life sustaining air bubble. Wreckage may also be ripped apart, causing further injury, death, or loss of victims. If this procedure is done, strong points of the aircraft such as the wings near their attachment to the fuselage should be used. If available, straps should be used since they are less likely to cut through the aircraft's structure.

Helicopter Crashes. In general, helicopter accidents should be handled in the same manner as fixed-wing crashes. As stated earlier, the location of fuel tanks (under the cabin floor) and the vertical nature of many chopper accidents increase fire danger. Use of EMS helicopters on emergency scenes creates the possibility that rescue personnel may actually be present when a mishap occurs. Such an event would place persons in the area in extreme danger since the crash and immediate postcrash events pose multiple hazards. The first response should be to seek cover since helicopter accidents characteristically cause a great deal of shrapnel to be thrown great distances at high speed. Once this hazard diminishes, persons should use extreme caution in approaching the aircraft. Even without fire, try to approach from upwind and uphill to reduce exposure to potential heat, smoke, or leaking fuel.

Because helicopter engines are usually located in the better protected mid-upper fuselage, they may remain running after the crash. Crew injuries or aircraft damage may prevent immediate shutdown. Due to damage to the rotors and/or the landing gear, the rotor blades may dip to unusually low attitudes, making approach extremely hazardous. Ideally, rescuers should wait for the engine and rotors to stop. If this is not possible, the rotor arc should be carefully surveyed and approached at a point of safe clearance (crawling if necessary). If the rotors are striking the ground it may cause the entire craft to wallow and roll (in addition to flying debris)—making a safe approach impossible. Attempt to approach on the opposite side of the aircraft from where the rotors are contacting the ground. If the pilot is disabled rescuers may have to shut down the engine(s). It is important for personnel to know engine shutdown procedures for common EMS aircraft. The fire suppression control handles or the fuel valve switches are generally the easiest methods of engine shutdown on many EMS type helicopters. Rescue crews should also be familiar with emergency equipment and exits on aircraft they work with.

Assisting the Post-Accident Investigation

Once patient care/extrication activities have been accomplished and hazards controlled, attention should turn to continued scene preservation and assisting the crash investigation. Confirm that proper aviation authorities have been notified and are en route. See that arrangements are made to meet and transport these officials to the site. Strict security of the entire accident scene, all wreckage and impact damage should be maintained. All unnecessary personnel should be kept out of the area—including the media and others who do not have an immediate function. This may be a very complicated task if wreckage is scattered over a wide area. Try to record any temporary evidence (ice, snow, soot, or impact marks) that may disappear or become altered. Photographs may be the easiest and most accurate method to accomplish this. Names of witnesses and where they can be contacted (home and work) should be obtained for investigators. Witnesses should be encouraged to immediately write a detailed account of what they observed.

CONCLUSION

The special problems presented in this chapter suggest that the practice of medicine in the field is, at best, a very inexact science. You may be left to your own wits to try to salvage what is best in a bad situation. Preparation and a plan, combined with field experience, can be of great assistance to the EMT who is faced with environmental hazards, mass casualties, or both. The information provided in this chapter is, by necessity, an overview, but it is worth reviewing from time to time to maintain a level of preparation.

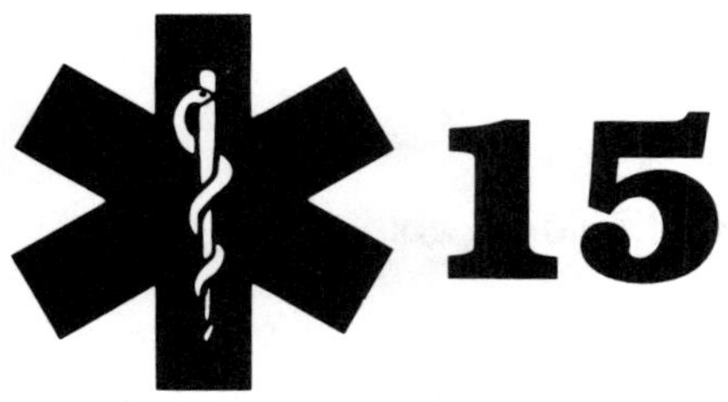

Medicolegal Aspects of Prehospital Care

INTRODUCTION

Most health care providers have a skeptical view of the legal system as it relates to their care and treatment of patients—fatalistic because most believe that a lawsuit against them or their organization will happen if they see enough patients, and realistic because it is true. Recent surveys show that approximately one claim will arise per 24,000 calls. In the prehospital care phase, this number is probably far under the actual number of claims, but it is impressive that most prehospital care providers will become involved in a lawsuit. This chapter presents a practical view of the legal system as it relates to prehospital care provider liability. You are a potential witness in a lawsuit either as a fact witness or as a defendant in an action arising from care rendered.

The framework of the typical lawsuit is described, with a focus on areas which present common challenges. You must recognize that there is an infinite variety of factual differences in specific cases and that state and local statutes and case law vary considerably. The intent of the following material is to educate, not to provide specific legal advice. The general term "provider" in the context of this chapter means any health care provider rendering care in the prehospital care phase.

OBJECTIVES

At the conclusion of this chapter, you should be able to:

1. Describe the basic principles of the criminal and civil legal system.
2. Define the negligence theory and explain how it relates to provision of prehospital care.
3. List various standard-of-care considerations which relate to prehospital providers.
4. Explain the importance of documentation and proper communication in the prehospital phase and how they protect both patient and provider.

COMMON LEGAL TERMS

The following glossary should be useful in understanding the basic legal system.

- *Complaint:* the initial pleading filed with the court in a medical malpractice action.
- *Plaintiff:* the person or party, usually the patient or his or her representative, who files a malpractice action.
- *Defendant:* the person or party, usually the provider or his or her employer, who is sued by the plaintiff.
- *Deposition:* testimony of any witness in a lawsuit taken before trial under oath in writing or by video.
- *Evidence:* any type of proof legally presented at trial through witnesses, records, documents, or objects to prove or disprove allegations.
- *Negligence:* the omission to do something which a reasonable person, guided by ordinary considerations which commonly regulate human affairs, would do or the commission of something which a reasonable or prudent person would not do.
- *Res ipsa loquitur:* literally, "the thing speaks for itself," meaning no expert is necessary to establish a standard-of-care deviation.
- *Subpoena:* an order from the court which requires a person to appear and testify at a particular time and place.

- *Statute of limitations:* time within which a legal action may be brought by a plaintiff in a civil case and not be barred.
- *Verdict:* the jury's decision with respect to matters of fact in issue.

THE LEGAL SYSTEM

The legal system is civilized society's mechanism to provide for orderly resolution of disputes and promote social order. Unfortunately, many of our patients are settling their disputes by means of bullets or blows. A lawsuit is essentially a paper bullet filed in a court of law which seeks through the legal system to right alleged wrongs. The law is broadly divided into two classifications, criminal and civil, which form the basis of rules governing people's actions.

Criminal Law

Criminal law deals with intentionally committed acts that are harmful to society. Criminal statutes are written by lawmakers who are part of a governing body. A person who violates and is found guilty of a crime pays a fine to the governing body or is placed in jail for a period of time. The person initiating the legal action in a criminal case is the governmental body; the person sued is the alleged lawbreaker. Proof of each element in a criminal case is based on a test of whether the evidence presented to the court is in favor of the plaintiff "beyond a reasonable doubt." Typical criminal laws involve assault and battery, rape, murder, child abuse, driving under the influence of alcohol, and drug peddling. Enforcement of criminal law involves governmental agencies with which prehospital care providers interact daily. Ignorance of the law is not excuse for failing to maintain evidence of criminal activity. You should be well advised to know directives within laws and their jurisdictions as they apply to reporting crimes.

Civil Law

Civil law involves disputes between persons and is the general area of law which governs medical malpractice lawsuits. "Medical malpractice" is a recognized phrase which is used to describe any conduct by a health care provider which, if faulty, produces liability. A person who has committed medical malpractice in the context of prehospital care is judged by the general standards of the community. These standards are derived from evidence which is found in statutes and in rules and regulations, but most often they are established by expert witnesses who testify whether or not the defendant has breached the standard of care in rendering emergency medical care to a patient. This area of law, as opposed to criminal law, deals with nonintentional torts; that is, the provider did not intend to harm the patient, but allegedly, harm occurred from the negligent conduct.

THE NEGLIGENCE THEORY OF LIABILITY

Within medical malpractice law, negligence is the primary theory of liability. Negligence has been defined as conduct which falls below the standard established by law for the protection of others against unreasonable risk of harm. In order to recover for negligent medical practice, the plaintiff must establish:

1. A duty of care was owed by the provider to the patient.
2. The provider violated the applicable standard of care.
3. The patient suffered damage.
4. The damage was proximately caused by the substandard care of the provider.

To establish these elements in a civil lawsuit against a health care provider, valid evidence must be presented to the fact-finder (jury). In a civil case, evidence is considered valid if it "more probably than not" occurred. This test of validity is not as heavy as that in criminal actions, where guilt must be established "beyond a reasonable doubt." If a judgment is entered against a provider in a civil lawsuit, money damages are awarded, as opposed to fines or imprisonment in the criminal law setting. This chapter places emphasis on the duty of providing care, as well as on the standard-of-care aspect, in accordance with the negligence theory of liability.

One of the more interesting rules of civil law involves the time frame within which medical malpractice lawsuits may be brought. Subject to certain exceptions, in most states, the plaintiff can bring a suit against a defendant up to a year after the alleged wrong, at a minimum, and it is important to recognize that if the plaintiff is a minor or incapacitated mentally, the statute of limitations never cuts off the right to sue. Generally, the incident that creates the basis for a lawsuit occurs a year or more before the lawsuit itself comes about. The provider has probably seen and treated literally hundreds of patients between the time of the event and the time when he or she is called upon to give a deposition or be a witness in a trial setting. Because of this time delay, the importance of well documented records is obvious.

DUTY

(Provider ⟶ duty ⟶ patient)

In the context of prehospital care, the duty of caring for a patient arises when you first establish contact with the patient and that contact is consented to. The duty arises because of your status as defined by statutes and regulations. Once a relationship with a patient is established, you the provider—whether a first responder, EMT, or EMT-paramedic—have a duty to act reasonably given the situation and your background, training, and experience.

CONSENT

When you first come in contact with a patient, the duty to act must begin with the establishment of consent for treatment. In general, consent is the mechanism through which you legally obtain permission to care for a patient with whom you come in contact. The important types of consent are:

Express Consent: A competent patient agrees by voice or writing to accept your care.

Implied Consent: A competent or incompetent patient is understood by law to have given his or her acceptance for treatment because of the factual situation.

Informed Consent: A competent patient has the right to know what treatments are planned and the risks involved in said treatments before giving express consent.

The consent issue generally is not a problem in prehospital care when the patient has a real or apparent life-threatening injury or illness. The patient, relative, or bystander has called for care, and when you arrive on the scene, offered care is not rejected; therefore, consent is implied. Problems do arise when providers arrive at a scene and are faced with a patient who does not agree to transport because of factors which may not be entirely clear: drug and alcohol ingestion, head injury, or psychiatric conditions. Your duty to evaluate the patient, though not expressly consented to, still exists. You should assess the situation as completely as possible, call for advice from medical control if necessary, and rely upon law enforcement officers to protect the patient from him or herself by protective custody (or arrest if necessary), if you reasonably believe that the patient is in a potentially life-threatening situation. In situations of doubt, you should always err on the side of action rather than inaction where a situation of no consent or refusal of consent exists, since it is very difficult to obtain all applicable facts at the scene.

The incompetent patient cannot give consent; a minor is considered incompetent in most situations. A situation can arise when parents cannot give express consent or will not give express consent for treatment of a child. When faced with this situation, other adults in charge of the child can give consent, and treatment and transport can generally be accomplished by operation of implied consent. Again, if you err on the side of preserving the life of the child, it is most appropriate to quickly notify law enforcement officers if transport cannot be accomplished with cooperation. You should not bodily move any incompetent patient against his or her will or the will of the parent/guardian until law enforcement authorities are part of the decision process.

Refusal of consent to treat and transport is not uncommon. After evaluation of the situation, if you determine the patient is competent to refuse treatment and/or transport, it is reasonable to obtain the patient's signature on a form indicating the patient acknowledges the refusal of care. More importantly, documentation of the situation by the provider, with names of witnesses recorded and an explanation of the circumstances of the refusal, will be evidence that you assessed the situation properly.

The law is generally on the side of the provider in the field, mandating that care be rendered rather than not rendered. If you're in doubt regarding the patient's capacity to give consent, and the situation involves a possibly unstable condition, treat and transport the patient since the risk of not doing so far outweighs the technicality of violating consent and being guilty of battery. Once you've established the provider/patient relationship, continue care until the patient is turned over to another provider of the same or higher level, or until care is no longer needed. Not to continue care when care is justified or potentially justified is abandonment and can be a deviation from the standard of care.

STANDARD-OF-CARE CONSIDERATIONS

(Duty ——→ Standard of Care)

The duty of the prehospital care provider to act is governed by the standard of care applicable to that level of provider. The first responder may or may not have a certification and licensure by the state; EMT and EMT-paramedic level providers generally must have certification and/or licensure by the governing body of the state in order to be able to legally provide care. It is through such licensure that providers in this setting are empowered to carry out the emergency medical care of patients suffering from medical and traumatic emergencies. In performing any medical evaluation or treatment, their actions are seen as extensions of a physician's actions. Standard-of-care considerations apply to all behavior of providers in the prehospital care phase, whether the action is derived directly from physician order or is an independent act.

Standard-of-care relative to providers in the prehospital care setting is based upon two broad areas: first, there are laws and regulations specifically delineating certain actions that can be carried out in the field. To not follow these rules as specified creates a near automatic presumption that the provider violated the standard of care applicable to his level of training. In addition, the prevalence of courses which are recognized throughout most states (for example: EMT, BTLS, ATLS, BCLS, and ACLS) serves to give providers standards of conduct given a particular patient presentation. Second, the standard of care in negligence cases is established by testimony from qualified witnesses who can speak for the skill expected of a provider in the same class as the accused and who answer questions of fact appropriate to the patient–provider encounter being reviewed. The witness in this situation is generally of the same background, training, and experience as the provider who is being evaluated. If there is an alleged standard-of-care deviation by a provider, the expert witness generally must state that this is a deviation in order for a medical malpractice action to survive unless the judge decides that lay people (in other words, a jury) can make the determination. This is often referred to as a *res ipsa* situation.

The Good Samaritan Statute

In most states, negligent conduct in the prehospital care environment may be excused by the mechanism of "Good Samaritan" statutes. The logic underlying the passage of these statutes is to encourage volunteer first aid in emergency situations outside the hospital environment. Typically, the law relieves the volunteer of all but gross negligence in his actions as long as they conform to his level of training in health care. A passer-by who sees a person in distress is under only a moral obligation to render care. Another key element of most Good Samaritan laws is that the care is rendered by a provider who does not already have a duty to act, that is, who is a true unpaid volunteer. Although some states may see the first responder as covered by the Good Samaritan law, it is strongly arguable that no providers in the prehospital care area can be protected by these statutes. Providers in this setting are not mere passers-by; they arrive at the scene because they are called and were on duty awaiting such calls. If you are off duty, however, you could be covered by the Good Samaritan protection as would any other professional, if the situation is emergent and if you render care which is unpaid and within your level of expertise.

Other Standard-of-Care Considerations

The conduct of providers as it relates to criminal law should be similar to the conduct of any lay person on the street, modified to the extent that providers find themselves in an aid-giving situation. To interfere with officers who are gathering evidence invites dispute; however, you should remember that the provider in the prehospital care environment owes a duty to evaluate the patient in accordance with standard emergency medical care practice. Interference by police in the treatment of accident victims should not occur; however, you should never interfere with police or other officers but should insist that adequate evaluation of patients be allowed as soon as possible regardless of evidence-gathering or other constraints. Often, medical evaluation and treatment is delayed, but mechanisms should be in place so that significant delays will not occur. You should stand by, record data, and render aid as soon as possible.

Standard-of-care questions involving who is in charge often arise at scenes of accidents or illness. Generally speaking, the person with the most advanced training is the person who has the authority to direct care. The EMT derives his or her medical authority and orders from protocols generated by the medical authority or medical director and from directions from a physician at a base station. Although physicians and nurses who stop at accident scenes are higher ranking and sometimes helpful, they can cause confusion and sometimes unwittingly delay treatment of patients. It is mandatory that providers cooperate and work together for the best interest of the patient, and no dispute should interfere with care. If there is a physican at the site of an injury or illness who assumes medical control, it is correct to strongly suggest that he or she continue medical control until the patient is transferred to another physician, if the situation warrants a physician's continued presence. Sometimes it is helpful to allow telephone communications with the medical control to be handled by the volunteer provider.

A question which often arises in the prehospital care area involves where to transport the patient. If the patient is alert and competent, then his or her wishes as to the admitting facility should generally be followed. Likewise, if the patient is medically stable, although not competent to choose a facility, the family's preference should be followed. Most often, this process will place the patient in the hands of physicians who know him or her.

A more complex question arises when a patient is not competent to make a decision with regard to the admitting facility or, in another instance, when the patient is deteriorating and needs to be stabilized at a closer or more appropriate facility than the one requested by the patient or family. Generally, you are well advised to use your best medical judgment in instances where there are alternative hospitals to take patients. Involved in that decision-making process are a number of factors, notably the presence of designated trauma centers. It is desirable to have in place transport protocols which handle the questions of who should be taken where. In the absence of such protocols, the ambulance services and providers should communicate regularly to determine availability of facilities for various types of patients.

The use of air transport to major medical centers has become increasingly prevalent. Providers who request air transport must know the types of patient situations which call for such transport, the means of securing the service, and proper precautions required when dealing with the mechanics of stabilizing patients, moving patients to the landing site, and loading patients. As with all patient transfers, appropriate documentation is mandatory.

The quantity of equipment involved in prehospital care is staggering. Statutes and regulations often address specifically what should be present in an ambulance certified by the state. Not to have an ambulance so equipped is generally seen as an automatic standard-of-care deviation. Likewise, not to have equipment in proper working order with documentation on quality control mechanical checks is inappropriate.

DOCUMENTATION AND REPORTING

Documentation and reporting are key elements in the prehospital care phase to insure that patients receive quality care. The written record involving the patient from beginning of treatment through the transfer to the emergency department of the hospital or another health care provider represents most of what you will remember months or years after the event if the care is reviewed for any reason. More importantly, however, the written record generated at the time of care and treatment focuses on problems, trends in vital signs, and times and types of emergency medical care administered. This information must be given to the next provider in line so that appropriate diagnostic and treatment decisions may be made. Most services have forms with multiple blanks which should be filled out consistently and completely; otherwise, the provider can be accused of not conforming to the acceptable standard of care.

State laws mandate in many situations the reporting of possible crimes and/or public health concerns. Such areas include any crime involving assault and battery, as well as suspected child abuse, communicable diseases, and animal bites. In general, you should report these types of patients to the providers in the emergency department for their evaluation of the situation and communication to governmental agencies involved. Confidentiality of records and information known about patients is based upon statutory considerations as well as the right of privacy and medical ethics. Although the physical records of a patient are the property of you or your employer, the *content* of the record can be examined by the patient or his or her representative, copied and used as evidence in any legal proceeding. Charting should be clear and concise and should be done as close to the time of the event as reasonably possible. Records which have been altered at a later date are usually indicators of substandard care or of your afterthoughts meant to help you and not the patient. If a record does need modification, make the correction by clear interlineation (not erasure) with appropriately dated and timed entries indicating the change(s). Or, better yet, attach a separate page to the record with the corrections to the original.

DAMAGES

If it can be proved that a provider had a duty to act and breached that duty by deviating from the established standard of care, then damages may be established in the court proceeding. This part of the medical malpractice lawsuit is accomplished by evidence which links the standard-of-care deviation to the patient's alleged damages. The four elements of a medical malpractice lawsuit are therefore tied together:

Causation
(Duty ——→ Standard-of-Care Breach ————→ Damages)

Providers are often faced with situations involving patients with devastating injuries and conditions incompatible with life. If, for example, a patient has undisputed signs at the scene of brain death, and the patient also has an unstable fractured neck, it most certainly would be a standard-of-care deviation not to stabilize the patient's neck in transport. However, in this hypothetical case, the plaintiff would certainly have a problem carrying the burden of proof of showing that the substandard care caused or contributed to the patient's death.

In the setting of any patient who has a sign of life, it is the standard of care to resuscitate first and reflect upon chances of survival later, rather than make any hasty decisions in the field regarding viability. Once begun, resuscitation should only be ended on order of a physician. You are well advised to render standard, aggressive care at all times once the decision is made to render care.

LIABILITY COVERAGE

If you are involved in a malpractice action, you will generally be protected by your employer as long as your actions took place within the normal scope of your employment and as long as your conduct conformed to what is reasonably covered and expected under the job description. Hypothetically, you might be sued individually for negligent actions during your employment, and the employer (or his or her insurance company) might have the option to protect or not protect you. In general, employers do provide coverage because of the relationship between employer and employee under the law of agency. However, you should not assume that you are guaranteed coverage if individually named in a lawsuit. For this reason, many providers purchase individual coverage for the possible legal exposure if sued individually and not protected by their employer. The decision to purchase individual malpractice coverage should be made on the basis of the contractual relationship between you and your employer and on the basis of other considerations, including availability of insurance, potential exposure, and cost.

CONCLUSION

You are compelled by the nature of your job to understand the legal system as it relates to the care and treatment of patients. The focus should be on providing good quality care which meets standards applicable to your level of expertise. Although lawsuits in the health care area are commonplace, the first responder, EMT or EMT-paramedic can minimize his or her exposure by properly communicating and documenting both the initial evaluation and the type of care administered.

Index

A

R

S

T

U

V

W